SAG

NATURE'S REMEDIES

SAGE

Nature's Remedy for the Third Age

Penelope Ody, MNIMH

SOUVENIR PRESS

First published 2000 by
Souvenir Press Ltd.,
43 Great Russell Street, London WC1B 3PA

ISBN 0 285 63555 7

Typeset by Rowland Phototypesetting Ltd,
Bury St Edmunds, Suffolk

Printed in Great Britain by
The Guernsey Press Co. Ltd.,
Guernsey, Channel Islands

Sage is warm without acrimony, most friendly to
the brain, grateful to the stomach preventing
coldness, flatulencies and indigestion there, and
giving a constantly and moderate never voracious
appetite, curing also a numbness, deafness,
dimness of sight and dullness of apprehension.
John Hill, *The Virtues of Sage*, 1763

Contra vim mortis
crescit salvia in hortis.
Cur moriatur homo
cui salvia crescit in horto?
(Against the power of death sage grows in the garden.
Why should a man die while sage grows in his garden?)
Roman proverb

The juice of sage drank with vinegar, has been of
good use in case of plague at all times.
Nicholas Culpeper, 1653

Sage helps the nerves and by its powerful might
Palsy is cured and fever put to flight.
Old French saying

Note to Readers

The aim of this book is to provide information on the uses of sage in the treatment of relevant diseases. Although every care has been taken to ensure that the advice is accurate and practical, it is not intended to be a guide to self-diagnosis and self-treatment. Where health is concerned—and in particular a serious problem of any kind—it must be stressed that there is no substitute for seeking advice from a qualified medical or herbal practitioner. All persistent symptoms, of whatever nature, may have underlying causes that need, and should not be treated without, professional elucidation and evaluation.

It is therefore very important, if you are considering trying sage for medicinal purposes, to consult your practitioner first, and if you are already taking any prescribed medication, do not stop it.

The Publisher makes no representation, express or implied, with regard to the accuracy of the information contained in this book, and legal responsibility or liability cannot be accepted by the Author or the Publisher for any errors or omissions that may be made or for any loss, damage, injury or problems suffered or in any way arising from following the advice offered in these pages.

Contents

Preface

This book is intended as an introduction to some of the impressive healing plants in the sage or *Salvia* family. The most familiar is, of course, common or broad-leaved sage, grown in many kitchen gardens, but there are plenty of others: Spanish or narrow-leaved sage, Greek sage which is so often confused with common sage, clary or the Chinese red sage now available in the West.

For generations, common sage was associated with health and a long life, with well-known country rhymes hinting at the longevity and well-being that come from eating it. Such traditions have tended to be dismissed by the orthodox medical profession as old wives' tales, but in sage's case modern research has shown that it can not only help to slow the steady progression of Alzheimer's disease, but also acts as a powerful antioxidant to combat damage and decay of the body's cells. Sage is also strongly oestrogenic, so is an ideal menopausal tonic.

Not all sage's powerful constituents are quite so friendly. Some—mainly thujones—are very toxic. The oil can be particularly damaging and, like all powerful herbs, sage needs to be treated with respect. It can be used safely at home for minor self-limiting ailments, but for more serious or chronic conditions professional help, ideally from a qualified medical herbalist, is essential. If you do intend using some of the self-help suggestions in this book then do so in consultation with your health care professional and do not simply replace prescribed medicines with the sage remedies suggested.

There is a great deal of confusion between sage species in commercially available products, so take great care with extracts purporting to be made only from less toxic Spanish or Greek sage.

Penelope Ody
December 1999

CHAPTER 1

Introducing Sage

Common sage, the herb most people associate with little more than stuffing for the Christmas turkey, is one of our most valuable medicinal herbs. Since ancient times it has been regarded as a sacred plant—the *herba sacra* of the Romans; the *salvia salvatrix* (sage the Saviour) of the mediaeval medical school at Salerno.

Sage was not only considered an essential cure-all for a wide array of everyday ailments, but was credited with the gift of longevity—a guarantee of a long and healthy life.

Throughout the Middle Ages this enthusiasm for sage continued, with writers declaring that 'the desire of sage is to render man immortal'. It was the final remedy: 'When a baby is given up for lost by the doctor, and nobody understands the illness which is going to take its life, prepare a decoction of sage and administer a small spoonful every five minutes; you will witness the resurrection of the infant . . .' (Palaiseul, 1973).

Sage was a favourite ingredient in many of the 'elixirs of life' popular throughout the Middle Ages, and its reputation as a longevity remedy continued well into modern times. In the early 1760s, the London physician John Hill produced a slim monograph entitled *The Virtues of Sage in lengthening human life with Rules to attain Old Age in Health and Chearfulness* [sic]. Over the course of some forty pages he details his common-sense approach to ageing:

Chearfulness promotes long life . . . to assist medicine in prolonging life the old man must avoid equally fatigue of mind and body but by no means extend this rule to the banishing of either exercise or thought . . .

... he will never live his natural time who does not know
the rule of moderation ... anger wastes the frame ...
... to live at ease is what he has to wish and to sum up all
to live at ease is the sure method to live long.

Sage, Hill tells us, is an important component in this simple
recipe—it 'continues health, preserves the faculties and memory,
and by a grateful warmth cheers, revives, refreshes and recruits'.
Yet, he goes on to ask, why were so many of his patients who
used sage no healthier than those who did not? Sage was regularly
eaten in May on bread and butter, taken in teas or mixed with
cheeses. But his patients who did so were no more likely to live
long lives than those who did not.

Hill concluded that it was because the leaves of sage were
used: 'but 'tis not in the leaves of plants that their principal
virtues reside, the roots and seeds in general possess the greatest
powers.'

So, in the true spirit of eighteenth-century scientific enquiry,
John Hill set up a series of experiments making extracts of sage
seeds, roots, leaves and flowers, gathered at different times of year
from his garden in Bayswater.

He concluded that red sage had the greatest virtue—although
his assessment of 'virtue' seemed to be based largely on which
extract smelt the most potent—and that the leaves were best when
gathered before flowering (in May): 'lightly cordial, strengthening,
stomachic'. Root extracts proved a dismal failure, although the
seeds were 'warm and cordial beyond the leaves, carminative and
friendly to the nerves'.

But John Hill still wasn't happy: none of his extracts seemed
to him to display the powers one might expect from such a reputed
elixir of life. So he began focusing on the aromatic aspects of
sage, gathering his herb in July when the flowers began to open:
'There is in their cups a fragrant resin of this kind, highly
flavoured, balmy, delicate and to the taste one of the most delicious
cordials that can be thought; warm and aromatic without
acrimony.'

Further experiments with a variety of alcohol and water mixtures convinced Hill that a 33 per cent alcoholic extract was the best, and that the plant had to be gathered at the exact moment when the flowers began to open, since 'certain juices are contained in or secreted from particular plants at certain seasons which do not exist in the same at other seasons'. Sage, he insisted, held its magic powers only at this particular time in July and the leaves, gathered in May, were a poor second best.

Whatever the merits of John Hill's careful experiments, sage has continued to be associated with curing the ailments of old age. Today it is being studied as a possible treatment for Alzheimer's disease, with early work suggesting that it can effectively slow down the rate of mental deterioration. It finds a role in the treatment of Parkinson's disease, although officially not as folk tradition would suggest, as a remedy to ease 'tremblings' in the limbs, but because it reduces the body's secretions so is helpful for controlling excess production of saliva which can be a significant discomfort for sufferers.

As a digestive remedy sage deserves far greater culinary use than in that occasional sage and onion stuffing: it is carminative to ease flatulence and indigestion, a bitter to stimulate the appetite and digestive function, and a warming, astringent remedy to combat stomach chills and diarrhoea.

The Romans believed that not only would sage prolong life, but could create it as well: they used the herb as a fertility tonic to encourage conception. It is now known to be an effective oestrogen tonic, valuable for stimulating and normalising menstrual function and helpful at the menopause—although as a potent oestrogenic it inevitably found use as an abortifacient when administered inappropriately during pregnancy.

As well as prolonging life, sage was also known as a preservative—one reason why it was used by country housewives as a wrapping for their cheeses. Today it has been shown to be one of our most potent antioxidants, helping to preserve cells and prevent decay.

Common sage, along with some of its many relatives listed in the next chapter, has been used in simple household remedies since the earliest times. Not all its reputed properties have yet been confirmed by modern research, but given its acknowledged actions in treating Alzheimer's disease, menopausal problems and as an antioxidant, sage certainly deserves its description as 'nature's remedy for the third age'.

CHAPTER 2

All Sorts of Sage

Common garden sage (*Salvia officinalis*) is just one of the 900 or so members of the *Salvia* genus, many of which are so valuable medicinally. But even 'common garden sage' is rather more complex than its name suggests. Modern herbalists have traditionally preferred 'purple sage', a red-leaved form of the plant which is now classified as *Salvia officinalis* 'Purpurescens Group', although at one time it was regarded as quite a different species and was sometimes labelled as *Salvia haematodes** or *S. colorata*.

Adding to the over-all confusion is Greek sage, *Salvia fruticosa*, which is frequently mixed with commercial supplies of dried common sage and, equally often, sold as 'garden sage' by nurseries. The plants have been confusing herbalists for generations, with writers from Dioscorides to Culpeper trying to differentiate between the two.

The sages are members of the Labiatae or mint family, which is now more usually called the Lamiaceae family. Sage is thus very closely related to an impressive array of other medicinal and culinary herbs, including the mints, lavenders, thymes, deadnettles and rosemaries. Salvias account for around 15 per cent of all species in the Lamiaceae.

All plants in the family are characterised by a square cross-section of their plant stems and by flowers whose petals are fused into a two-lipped corolla (see diagram 1). Although sage flowers

---

* *S. haematodes* is the name of a garden ornamental which has lavender-blue flowers and a basal rosette of large, dark green, wavy-edged leaves. It is not used medicinally, although learned papers have detailed investigations of 'red sage (*S. haematodes*)'—presumably because the name suggests it has red leaves and is therefore the botanical name of purple-leaved forms of *S. officinalis*.

can seem to vary significantly, all have this basic fused structure. Pollination is characteristically by insects which brush against a sterile anther when entering the flower, thus triggering fertile anthers to sprinkle pollen on the insect's back, ready for transfer to the fertile style of a neighbouring flower.

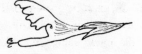

Diagram 1: Sage flowers.

Salvias are typically shrubs or perennials with very few true annuals, no trees and no climbers. Species range from popular garden flowers, such as the red-flowered *Salvia splendens*, to shrubs like *Salvia officinalis* or common sage, so widely used in European cooking and herbal medicine. Several other species have a long tradition of therapeutic use, including cancer weed (*S. lyrata*), used in Native American medicine, and *Dan Shen* (*S. miltiorrhiza*) one of Chinese medicine's most important tonic herbs (see chapter 7). Others are worth cultivating for their flavours or scents—pineapple sage (*S. elegans* 'Scarlet Pineapple') which adds a delicious flavour to ice-creams or sponge cakes, or blackcurrant sage (*S. microphylla* var. *microphylla*) which is equally tasty.

Among the more significant members of the *Salvia* genus are:

Jim sage (*S. clevelandii*)
Common name: blue sage

Description: evergreen shrub growing to around 60cm (24in) in height. The plant has hairy stems and wrinkled, aromatic leaves up to 2.5cm (1in) long. Blue-violet flowers in short whorls appear in summer.

Parts used: leaves

Jim Sage originates from California where Native Americans traditionally used the crushed mucilaginous seeds mixed in water as a coating to prevent evaporation of moisture from the mouth and throat during hot, dry weather (Vogel, 1970). Today the aromatic leaves are mainly added to pot pourri.

Tropical sage (*S. coccinea*)
Common name: Texas sage

Description: a perennial, usually grown in Europe as a half-hardy annual. It grows to around 1m (3ft) with an upright, branching habit. The hairy stems carry dark green hairy leaves with grey undersides, up to 6cm (2½in) long, varying from ovate to triangular in shape. *Coccinea* means scarlet and accurately describes the bright flower spikes borne in whorls up to 30cm (12in) long. Individual flowers are around 2cm (1in) long with a green or purple calyx. *S. coccinea* grows wild throughout Central and South America and the West Indies, although it is believed to be Mexican in origin.

Parts used: leaves

Although mainly grown as a garden ornamental, tropical sage is highly aromatic and the leaves make a useful addition to pot pourri.

Fruit-scented sage (*S. dorsiana*)
Common name: Honduras sage

Description: a tender perennial, *S. dorsiana* is a native of Honduras and rarely flowers in European climates. It is mainly grown in gardens for the fruity scent of its leaves—hence the name. The plant grows to around 1m (3ft), freely branching with an upright habit, lime-green ovate leaves up to 18cm (7in) in length with serrated margins. Both leaves and stems are very hairy. The flowers are magenta, up to 6cm (2½in) long in whorls on spike-like inflorescences up to 15cm (6in long).

Parts used: leaves

As the name suggests, the strongly smelling leaves make a useful addition to pot pourri or for flavouring soft drinks. They can also be chopped and added to cakes and salads or used to flavour salad dressings.

Pineapple sage (*S. elegans* 'Scarlet Pineapple'; also known as *S. rutilans*)

Description: this frost-tender perennial grows to around 1.5m (5ft) with hairy, ovate-lanceolate leaves, up to 10cm (4in) long, which have a strong pineapple scent. It has bright scarlet flowers in whorls on long (up to 20cm/8in) inflorescences which bloom from October until killed by frost. The plant can survive mild winters and will continue flowering through until January or February, but in British gardens is best grown in containers in greenhouse or conservatory.

Parts used: leaves

Originally from Mexico, pineapple sage is easily confused with its close relative tangerine sage (*S. elegans*)—the scent is clearly the obvious identifier. Pineapple sage is late-flowering and has been cultivated in Europe since 1873 (Sutton, 1999). The pine-apple-scented leaves are ideal for flavouring sponge cakes, soft drinks or fruit salads. They can also be chopped and added to meat dishes, such as gammon or pork, to give a pleasant sage/pineapple dressing (see p. 115).

Greek sage (*S. fruticosa*; also known as *S. triloba*, *S. cypria* or *S. libanotica*)
Common names: Turkish sage, Lebanese sage

Description: leaf shape varies from the ovate leaves of *S. officinalis* to pinnate forms, with some having one large terminal and two small lateral lobes—hence *triloba*. Flowers are very similar to *S. officinalis* but tend to be pink or mauve rather than blue, with a variable red or green calyx. Plants are shrubby, growing to around 60cm (24in) in height with a spread of about 1m (3ft). The charac-teristic lobed leaves are not always apparent, which adds to the confusion with *S. officinalis*.

Parts used: leaves. oil

S. fruticosa is used both as common sage and Spanish sage (see chapter 6) and grows throughout the eastern Mediterranean. As already noted (see p. 17), it is very easily confused with common sage and the dried leaves are a frequent adulterant to commercial supplies of *S. officinalis*—up to 95 per cent may be *S. fruticosa* (Mabberley, 1987).

Sage plants sold in nurseries and garden centres may also be *S. fruticosa* rather than *S. officinalis*, and since not all Greek sage leaves are characteristically trilobed it is not always easy to tell the difference. Greek sage leaves are smoother and narrower, while common sage leaves are broader.

The properties of these two species are fairly similar but their chemical compositions are quite different—which becomes significant when considering the essential oils extracted from the plant (chapter 6). Like common sage. Greek sage also contains toxic thujones (see chapter 4), although markedly less so than common sage, so it should be avoided by epileptics and in pregnancy.

S. fruticosa was well known to the ancient Greeks and has been identified on Cretan frescoes from around 2000 BC. The leaves are traditionally used in Cyprus to make a pleasant-tasting infusion known as *chanomilia*, while in Greece they are combined with *S. pomifera* to produce *faskomelo* tea.

Chia (*S. hispanica, S. polystachya, S. mexicana*, or *S. columbariae*)

Description: a number of South American varieties of sage are variously used to produce 'chia seeds'. These are all half-hardy plants, rarely found in Europe, although *S. polystachya* is listed in one of the UK National Collections of Salvias held at the Kingston Maurward College near Dorchester in Dorset. They tend to be vigorous, late-flowering sages, often growing to 3m (10ft) in height, with ovate leaves and blue to purple flowers.

Parts used: seeds

In Mexico the mucilaginous seeds are mixed with water, lemon juice and sugar to make a drink, while an oil extract is used in painting. Chia seeds are also used in many parts of South America in cooking, added to cakes and soups. They are sometimes used medicinally in North America and are said to be expectorant, demulcent and diaphoretic (Frawley and Lad, 1988), although few detailed reports of their use are available.

21

Judean sage (*S. judaica*)

Description: a herbaceous perennial with mid-green leaves up to 13cm (5in) long covered in short white hairs, making them very soft to the touch. The outer leaves of each cluster tend to have basal lobes while the main leaf shape can be very variable—from lyrate to oblong. Leaf edges are often wavy. Whorls of up to 20 flowers, which are small and vary from lilac to violet, appear from early summer to early autumn. The plant is regarded by some botanists as a subspecies of *S. verticillata* (whorled clary).

A native of Syria, Lebanon and Israel, this sort of sage, according to Exodus 37, was the origin of the seven-branched candlestick or Menora of Judaism. The symbol is based on the inflorescence of this particular species (Duke, 1983).

Spanish sage (*S. lavandulifolia*)
Common names: lavender-leaved sage, narrow-leaved sage

Description: evergreen shrub very similar to common sage, but with narrow, oblong, whitish-grey leaves which cluster around the base of the plant with almost leafless flowering stems. Many botanists regard it as a subspecies of *S. officinalis*, so closely are the two plants related. Plants are smaller than *S. officinalis*, reaching around 30cm (12in) in height. The leaves are up to 5cm (2in) long and have a rosemary- or camphor-like smell when crushed. The blue/purple flowers appear in early summer with around 6–8 blooms spread widely along the raceme. Native to mountainous areas of Spain, SW France and the Balkans.

Parts used: leaves, essential oil (see p. 77)

The leaves are often used as a substitute for *S. officinalis* and may contaminate commercial supplies depending on source. They are also widely used in the perfumery market and as a food flavouring. Like common sage, Spanish sage leaves are a popular folk remedy for digestive upsets, menstrual disorders, nervous upsets and depression. Although Spanish sage contains negligible amounts of toxic thujone (see chapter 4), it is advisable to avoid both the oil and high doses of the herb in pregnancy.

Cancer weed (*S. lyrata*)
Common names: wild sage, wild meadow sage

Description: when flowering *S. lyrata* grows to around 50cm (20in) in height, with basal leaves spreading up to 30cm (12in) in diameter. Leaves can be up to 20cm (8in) long and are usually described as lyrate (shaped like a lyre with a broad round terminal lobe and a pair of rounded lateral lobes)—hence the name. The leaves are dark green with maroon markings along the veins and leaf edges and may turn entirely maroon in dry weather. The plant flowers in early summer, with deep maroon stems carrying widely spaced whorls of violet/purple blooms up to 3cm (1½in) long.

Parts used: leaves, roots

S. lyrata is a native of the northern and central states of the USA and was used medicinally by various Native American people. The Catawbas on the East Coast, for example, used the roots in a salve for skin sores, while early settlers used the leaves on warts (Vogel, 1970).

Red bush (*S. microphylla* var. *microphylla*; also known as *S. grahamii*)
Common name: blackcurrant sage

Description: a shrub, not usually fully hardy, with variable leaf shapes which are generally ovate with finely toothed margins, 5cm (2in) long. Flowers are usually borne in whorls of two on racemes 10–20cm (4–8in) long, the upper lip being hooded with the larger lower lip widely spreading. Flowers can vary from crimson to pink depending on cultivar. In warm climates the bush will easily reach 3m (10ft).

Parts used: leaves, flowering tops

This sage is another which originates from Mexico and several cultivars are grown as garden ornamentals. One of the most popular is 'Kew Red' which grows to around 1.5m (5ft), with striking cherry-red flowers. *S. microphylla* var. *wislizenii* is a smaller-leaved, slightly hardier variety with magenta flowers. The leaves

23

and flowering tops are used in Mexico in infusions to treat fevers and digestive upsets.

Dan Shen (*S. miltiorrhiza*)
Common names: red sage, Chinese sage

Description: branched perennial growing to 60cm (2ft) in height. The stems are densely covered with hairs and the opposite leaves are divided into as many as seven ovate lobes up to 8cm (3in) long. Reddish-purple flowers are carried in whorls of possibly ten blooms on long racemes, up to 20cm (8in) long.

Parts used: root

The plant grows throughout China—just about everywhere from sunny mountains to roadside ditches. Commercial production is largely concentrated in the provinces of Sichuan and Shanxi.

Dan Shen is one of the more important Chinese medicinal herbs, mainly used for heart problems and gynaecological disorders (see chapter 7). The plant was given its Latin name by Alexander von Bunge (1803–90) in an 1833 publication, *miltiorrhiza* being derived from *miltos* meaning 'red lead' and *rhiza* for 'root'. Seeds first arrived in the West in the eighteenth century when the plant was cultivated in the Paris botanical garden. It is not a particularly showy member of the sage family so is rarely found outside botanical gardens or specialist plant collections.

In China the related species *S. przewalskii* or *S. przewalskii* var. *mandarinorum* (known as *Gansu Dan Shen*) and *S. bowleyana* (known as *Nan Dan Shen*) are used in similar ways to *Dan Shen*. They may also be sold under that name or be mixed with the main species (Yen, 1992). In Yunnan province, *S. yunnanensis* is used in folk medicine as a local alternative to *Dan Shen*, while *S. trijuga* and *S. plectranthoides* make similar alternatives in parts of Hubei, Shanxi, Sichuan, Xizang and Guizhou.

Kalijarri (*S. moorcroftiana*)
Common names: shobri, thut, gurgumna, papra

Description: the entire plant is hairy with long-stalked leaves, up to 25 × 15cm (10 × 6in), varying from ovate to lanceolate or oblong. The upper surfaces are grey-green with a white, very hairy underside. A single flowering stem produces whorls of pale lilac-blue flowers with a distinctive pair of pink bracts at the base of each whorl. The plant is not fully hardy and tends to behave more as a biennial, dying down after setting seed, than a true perennial.

Parts used: leaves, seeds

Kalijarri originates in the South Himalayas and is found growing wild from Afghanistan to Nepal, on slopes up to 2,800m (9,000ft) above sea level. The leaves are used in the Punjab for treating coughs, and as a vermifuge; included in poultices for boils, wounds and skin infections. The seeds are an emetic and are also given for dysentery and haemorrhoids (Ambastha, 1986). Several other species of sage are used in Indian folk medicine—seeds of *tukham malanga* (*S. aegyptiaca*), for example, are also used in the Punjab as a demulcent for diarrhoea and haemorrhoids (Ambastha, 1986; Singh *et al.*, 1983).

Common sage (*S. officinalis*)
Common names: garden sage, true sage, Dalmatian sage, *herba sacra*, broad-leaved sage, sawge, purple sage, red sage

Description: evergreen sub-shrub, growing up to 80cm (32in) in height from a woody base with a spread of around 1m (3ft). The leaves are soft, pale grey-green and oblong to elliptic up to 6cm (2½in) long; the undersides of the leaves are paler and more hairy. Deep blue or violet flowers, appearing in June and July, are borne in whorls of up to 20 on the flowering stem, with individual blooms that may be 2.5cm (1in) long. White or pink flowers also occur naturally from time to time and have been developed in a variety of cultivars.

Parts used: leaves, flowering tops, essential oil (see p. 80)

The plant is popular with bees and butterflies. Native to the Mediterranean, Balkans and North Africa, common sage is now grown worldwide; production is highest in Italy, Turkey and the USA. Commercial supplies are often adulterated by as much as 95 per cent with *S. fruticosa* or *S. lavandulifolia* (Mabberley, 1987).

There are numerous cultivars of *S. officinalis* including:

- *S. officinalis* 'Albiflora'—a white-flowered cultivar with the same grey-green leaves, popular with designers of white and silver gardens.
- *S. officinalis* 'Berggarten'—a low-growing variety (up to 40cm/16in high) with broader leaves and few flowers.
- *S. officinalis* 'Grete Stolze'—a mauve-flowered variant with more pointed, grey-green leaves.
- *S. officinalis* 'Icterina'—a yellow/gold variegated form, which seldom flowers, popular with herb garden designers. It tends to be less robust than other cultivars.
- *S. officinalis* 'Kew Gold'—a dwarf variety with bright yellow leaves, also popular with herb garden designers.
- *S. officinalis* Purpurescens Group—the purple sage or red sage which is often preferred by medical herbalists. The flowers are violet-purple and a number of cultivars (e.g. 'Purpurescens Variegata' and 'Robin Hill') can be found in specialist nurseries.
- *S. officinalis* 'Rosea'—a pink-flowered variant with the same grey-green leaves.
- *S. officinalis* 'Tricolor'—a very pretty ornamental variety with white, green and pink variegated leaves and mid-blue flowers, which is very aromatic and compact but less hardy than the original species. It is popular for container-growing but needs to be over-wintered in a cold frame.

Kakaburadi (*S. plebeia*)

Common names: *bhutulasi, jingiba, kammar kas, samundar, sokh, sathi*

Description: a hairy erect annual growing to 15–90cm (6–18in) in height, with mid-green ovate leaves. Flowers, which appear in the spring, are small and white, carried in whorls of 20–30 blooms on short racemes. It is found on river banks and roadsides through much of southern China and South-east Asia.

Parts used: whole plant, seeds

The whole plant is used throughout India as a diuretic and anthelmintic. The seeds, which are highly mucilaginous, are given as a remedy for diarrhoea, haemorrhoids and menorrhagia (Ambastha, 1986). In southern China, the plant is regarded as anti-inflammatory, antibiotic, diuretic, styptic and a blood purifier (Li, 1985). It is used for treating tonsillitis, mouth ulcers, kidney disorders and bronchitis, while externally it is recommended for mastitis, piles and vaginitis. Boiling the herb with pork to make a soup is a traditional Hong Kong treatment for tuberculosis.

Apple-bearing sage (*S. pomifera*)

Description: evergreen shrub with light green, wrinkled, velvety leaves similar in shape and texture to common sage. The plant grows to around 1m (3ft) in height. The violet-blue flowers are borne in whorls on branched racemes in early summer. It takes its name from the fleshy galls, produced by gall wasps, which appear on the stems.

Parts used: leaves, galls

The leaves are generally used as a substitute for *S. officinalis* in the Mediterranean areas where the plant grows wild, and in Greece it is combined with *S. fruticosa* (*q.v.*) to make a tea. The galls are candied as medicinal sweets and also made into a conserve.

Clary sage (*S. sclarea*)
Common names: clary, clary wort, common clary, clear eye, see bright, wild spinach, muscatel sage, Vatican sage

Description: a hardy perennial or biennial which may reach 120cm (4ft) in height, capable of spreading to 80cm (32in) in its first season. The plant has large, wrinkled, green/purplish ovate to oblong leaves, up to 2.5cm (1in) long, at the base of the plant. The pink/mauve flowers appear in June and July in whorls of as many as six blooms each, with a large flower bract; these persist after flowering is over so that the flower stems remain an attractive feature in the garden for months thereafter. Native to Southern Europe and South-west Asia, but now widely cultivated.

Parts used: leaves, flowers, seeds, oil

Although clary sage, with its origins in Southern Europe, thrives in hot sun and dry, chalky soil it is also very hardy and will survive a British winter quite happily. The plant is a bitter astringent with mucilaginous seeds and a distinctive balsam-like aroma.

The botanical name comes from the Latin *clarus*, meaning sight, and the seeds were once thought to help vision and clear grit from the eye. Its common name 'clary' is similarly derived from 'clear eye'. Inserting a seed into the eye encouraged mucilage to form, which enveloped the offending grit which could then be easily removed by an eye-bath.

The oil is popular in aromatherapy (see p. 83) and was once added to incense—hence the common name Vatican sage. Clary sage oil is also used in eau-de-Cologne, vermouth and liqueurs. The plant has a reputation for creating euphoria and it was formerly added to beer to enhance the alcoholic effect—or as Mrs Grieve (1931) quotes from Matthias l'Obel (1538-1616): 'Some brewers of Ale and Beere doe put it into their drinke to make it more heady, fit to please drunkards, who thereby, according to their several dispositions, become either dead drunke, or foolish drunke, or madde drunke . . .'

The leaves are also used medicinally—mainly as a digestive remedy to stimulate the appetite and combat nausea and vomiting.

Clary sage can be taken in teas for menstrual problems and the leaves have been used in folk medicine in poultices and compresses for minor wounds and sores.

Clary sage can also be combined with elderflowers and infused in Rhine wines to give a muscatel flavour—in Germany it is known as *muskateller salbei* from this long tradition of simulating true muscatel wine.

The flowers can be added to salads and the young leaves made into fritters or used in teas (chapter 9).

Wild clary (*S. verbenaca*)

Common names: vervain sage, wild English clary, vervain, Christ's eye, Oculus Christi

Description: a robust perennial growing to 50–75cm (20–30in), with dark green leaves, ovate to oblong, up to 10cm (4in) long and 7cm (3in) wide. The leaf edges are wavy and irregularly dentate, while the upper leaf surface is wrinkled with glandular hairs. Flowering stems are small with inflorescences carrying as many as 10 whorls, each with about six blooms, lavender to purple and around 1.5cm (½in) long, from midsummer to early autumn.

Parts used: leaves, seeds

A native of much of southern and eastern Britain, wild clary is one of only two native British sages (the other is *S. pratensis* or meadow sage). Like *S. sclarea*, wild clary seeds were used to remove foreign bodies from the eye, thanks to the thick coating of mucilage which rapidly develops. Traditionally wild clary was believed to be a more effective remedy than cultivated clary sage. Extracts were also believed to help strengthen the eyes, especially in the elderly, and were used to clear eye inflammations and improve the sight.

A decoction of the leaves was recommended by Culpeper as a digestive remedy and he also adds that this will 'scatter congealed blood in any part of the body'—a recommendation reminiscent of the Chinese use of *Dan Shen* (see chapter 7).

Painted sage (*S. viridis*)
Common names: bluebeard, red-topped sage, annual clary

Description: a true annual and native to much of Southern Europe, painted sage grows to around 60cm (24in) with branched stems, mid-green ovate or oblong leaves, and white, pink or purple flowers in whorls on long racemes. The flowers are quite small (1.5cm/ ½in) long but the calyces and papery bracts immediately below the flowers are distinctive and will persist until autumn, making the plant a useful addition to the flower garden.

Parts used: leaves, flowering spikes, seeds, oil

Painted sage was introduced into England in Elizabethan times and became a popular culinary herb. The plant is aromatic and antiseptic, and an infusion of leaves was traditionally used as a mouthwash for sore gums. The oil was used to flavour wine and beer.

CHAPTER 3

Sage—Myths and Mystery

He who would live for aye
Must eat sage in May

While the ancients reputedly asked, *Cur moriatur homo cui Salvia crescit in horto?* (Why should a man die while sage grows in his garden?), generations have recited the more familiar country rhyme above as a reminder of sage's association with longevity. Drinking sage tea may not have been a guarantee of a long and healthy life, as John Hill noted (see chapter 1), but it was certainly worth trying.

This association with longevity seems to have developed from sage's reputation as a cure-all and general prophylactic for a wide range of diseases rather than from any specific life-giving tradition. Indeed, the earliest surviving Western herbals make little mention of longevity or prophylactics, and often leave us uncertain as to which variety or varieties of sage they are describing.

The ancient Greeks identified two varieties of sage: *elelisphakos* (ελελισφακος), usually identified as Greek sage (*S. fruticosa*), and *sphakos* (σφακος) which many writers claim to be common sage (*S. officinalis*). The opposite may just as easily be true: Theophrastus, writing around 300 BC, suggests that the difference between the two plants is 'like that between cultivated and wild; for the leaf of *sphakos* is smoother, smaller and less succulent, while that of *elelisphakos* is rougher' (Hort, 1916). Given the variation in *S. fruticosa* leaves and their very close similarities with common sage, it is hardly a clear guide for differentiating between the two plants.

Pliny, usually a reasonable source of Greek and Roman herbal traditions, simply adds to the confusion by muddling Theophrastus' *sphakos* (οφακος) with the word for lentil (φακος), so we have his delightful description that:

There is a wild lentil called *elelisphacos* by the Greeks (*sphacos* by others), smoother then the cultivated lentil, with a smaller, drier and more scented leaf. There is also another kind of it wilder still and with a heavy smell. The other, the more cultivated variety, has leaves like those of a quince, but smaller and pale, which are boiled with the branches (Jones, 1951).

Dioscorides (*c*. AD 60) is equally vague, suggesting that *elelisphakos* is actually our *S. officinalis*—which, as the famous translation by John Goodyer (1655) continues: 'some call Elaphoboscon, some Sphagnon, some Ciosmin, some Phagnon, some Becion, ye Egyptians Apusi, the Romans Cosalon, others Salvia . . .'

The Grete Herbal, a 1526 translation of an earlier work known as *Circa Instans*, perpetuates Theophrastus' preoccupation with wild and cultivated forms of sage:

There be ii maners of it. The tame and the wylde; this is called eupatory . . . The tame conforteth more than the wylde but the wylde unstoppeth the pypes more than the tame and hath vertue in conforttynge synewes. The wyne that sawge is soden in is good for them that have the falling evyll.

However, William Turner—known as the 'father of English botany'—gives these arguments short shrift:

Dioscorides maketh but one kind of sage, but Theophrastus maketh two kinds . . . but now there are found more kinds, the which, though they differ one from another much in roughness and smoothness, in greatness and smallness, and in diversity of colours, yet in my judgement do agree in one virtue and property, and although some be stronger than other some be (1562).

A hundred years later, Nicholas Culpeper (1653) was still talking of two types of sage—the 'common garden sage' and 'sage of virtue'. His entry for common sage is very reminiscent of Turner's earlier herbal, but 'sage of virtue' he describes as 'frequently having two small pieces or ears growing on them next the stalk' which rather suggests Greek sage (see p. 20). He describes an infusion of this variety as:

> powerfully by sweat and urine and removes female obstructions. The expressed juice drank for a considerable time is excellent against rheumatic pains; and was formerly celebrated against venereal complaints but since the introduction of mercury into practice its use has been set aside.

Sage as cure-all

These early sources give little indication of any life-giving properties of sage when eaten in May—although they do provide plenty of therapeutic actions which continue to be repeated and extended in numerous herbals over the following centuries. Pliny tells us that:

> It promotes menstruation and urine, and heals the wounds of the stingray, numbing the region affected. It is also taken in drink with wormwood for dysentery. With wine it also brings on delayed menstruation, while a draught of its decoction checks any excess. The plant applied by itself staunches the blood of wounds. It also cures snake bite, and if boiled down in wine allays pruritis of the testicles. Our modern herbalists call this plant *elelisphacus* in Greek and *salvia* in Latin, a plant like mint, hoary and aromatic. An application brings away the dead unborn baby, as well as worms in sores and ears (Jones, 1951).

While Dioscorides says that:

> Ye decoction of the leaves and of ye branches hath the power being drank to move ye urine and ye menstrua and to draw

33

out ye embrya of ye *pastinaca marina* [a stinging fish]. It dyes ye hair black also and it is a wound herb and a blood stancher and a cleanser of ye wild ulcers. But ye decoction of ye leaves and of ye branches of them with wine being fomented assuageth ye itchings about ye privities. *Elelisphacon* dissolves chilliness, ye cough and it is good being taken with *Rosaceam* and *Cerat* [an ointment base made of rush extracts and beeswax] for all ye bad ulcers and being drank with white wine it cures ye paine of ye spleene and ye dysenterie. In like sort being given to drink, it cures blood spitters and is available for all cleansings of woman, but ye most wicked women making a pessum of it do apply it and cast out ye embrya (Goodyer, 1655)

The list of therapeutic virtues continued to grow, and by the sixteenth and seventeenth centuries sage was established as a cure for the stings of fish and serpents, a remedy both for falling sickness (epilepsy) and rheumatic or arthritic pains; notable as a diuretic, emmenagogue, styptic, vulnerary and anti-pruritic; a cough remedy suitable for chronic problems, such as bronchitis and consumption:

Orpheus saith that two cyats of the juice of sage with one ounce of honey, if it be given unto a man with drink fasting, will stop the spitting of blood; but it is good against the phthisic and exulceration of the lungs, if it be dressed thus: take spikenarde two drams of seed; of sage, parched, beaten and softed, fourteen drams; of pepper twelve drams. Meng all these together in the juice of the sage and make pills thereof, and give a dram at a time in the morning to the patient fasting, and so much against night, and drink water after the pills (Turner, 1562).

It was a popular gargle for sore throats: 'Gargles likewise are made with sage, rosemary, honey-suckle, and plantain, boiled in wine or water, with some honey or alum put thereto to wash sore mouths and throats, cankers or the secret parts of man or woman, as need require.' (Culpeper, 1653); and known as a warming remedy to combat 'cold humours': 'The sawce made of sawge, percely and vynegre with a lytell peper is good to conforte the appetye that is febled by colde humours in the stomake.' (*The Grete Herbal*).

A hot and dry herb

Combating 'cold' was an important tactic for physicians in the cooler climates of Northern Europe at a time when medical theory was still firmly rooted in the Galenic medicine of the ancient Greeks. They had believed that the world and all things in it were derived from four elements—earth, air, fire and water—and the intrinsic character of these elements in terms of hot or cold, damp or dry, was a prime influence. 'Humours'—related to these same elements and qualities—were produced in the body and determined not only health and disease but also personality and character: too much cold and dampness led to the 'phlegmatic' man, likely to suffer from watery catarrh and with a tendency for slow thinking, while the hot and dry 'choleretic' was prone to inflammations, with a hot temper to match (see diagram 2).

Herbs were also categorised as hot and cold, dry or damp, in the same way. The medieval *Tacuinum Sanitatis* considered sage

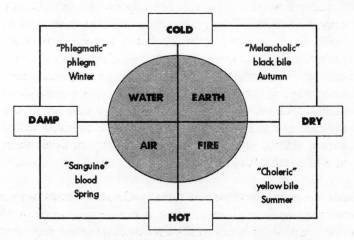

Diagram 2: The Galenic model relating humours and elements.

to be 'warm in the first degree and cold in the second' and *The Grete Herbal* agrees: 'Sawge is hote in the first degree and drye in the second'.

Three centuries later, Turner (1562) quotes Galen as declaring the plant 'of an evident hot complexion and something binding'— the binding or astringent activity being synonymous with dryness. He goes on: 'the heating power of sage is evidently known, but the binding virtue is but small.' A few years later Gerard (1597) similarly plays down the dryness: 'manifestly hot and drie in the beginning of the third degree.'

By Culpeper's day there were different priorities: 'Jupiter claims this,' he says, 'and bids me tell you it is good for the liver, and to breed blood'—although he then goes on to repeat Turner's list of therapeutics rather than launching on some hitherto neglected attributes. Perhaps he was thinking of *Dan Shen*?

Hidden well-being

Yet despite sage's comprehensive range of therapeutic properties—not untypical of the catalogue of virtues ascribed to many other herbs in those days—there must have been more to this plant than met the official chronicler's eye. The name *salvia* is variously said to derive from the Latin *salvere*, to be well or to be saved, *salveo*, I heal or save, or *salvus*, well-being. This became corrupted to *sauja* or *sauge* (the French name) and hence Middle English *sawge* and *sage*. It was also known in the Middle Ages as *herba sacra*, the holy herb, and *herbe sacrée* remains a common French country name for the plant. To the tenth-century physicians at Europe's first medical school in Salerno, sage was known as *salvia salvatrix* or 'sage the saviour'.

By the Middle Ages sage's links with a long and healthy life were clearly well established and the old Roman proverb is paraphrased in the twelfth-century *Macer's Herbal* (Sinclair Rohde, 1922) as:

> Why of seknesse deyeth man
> Whill sawge in gardeyn he may han.

The fourteenth-century writings of the Physicians of Myddfai also contain references to sage's prophylactic qualities. These Welsh manuscripts are of mixed parentage, and while it is nice to believe that they provide an insight into Celtic medicine, they are largely based on the same conventional Greek and Arabic sources used by later authors like William Turner and John Gerard. The currently available edition of the Myddfai texts is a translation from Welsh published by John Pughe in 1861 and is drawn from *The Red Book of Hergest* (*c*. 1400) and the *Book of Howel the Physician*—now regarded as an early nineteenth-century fake produced by lolo Morgannwg, a well-known forger (Fox, 1999), which successfully duped Mr Pughe.

Authentic or not, the Myddfai material lists some 'Virtues of Sage' reminiscent of Dioscorides and Pliny, and the entry concludes with a tonic recipe for preserving health:

> Let some thereof be taken, pounded small, and the juice mixed with white wine, strong wort, or old mead for a night and then strained, then drank fasting. By God's help it will cure the patient. It is a good thing for those in health to drink half a draught in the morning fasting of this potion, in order to preserve health (Pughe, 1861).

Belief in sage as a health-giving longevity remedy was still prevalent in the eighteenth century when John Hill wrote his enthusiastic monograph (chapter 1) and evidence of its widespread use as a household standby also comes from John Quincy's *Complete English Dispensatory* (1724). He mentions two sorts of sage—*Salvia major* 'most in use in the Shops', which he describes as being 'red or green', and '*Salvia minor* or *angustifolia*' which is 'not used in the Shops but much in private Families under the names Sage of Virtue and Tea-Sage.' *Salvia major*, judging by Gerard's more detailed descriptions, is *S. officinalis*, while *S. minor* is reminiscent of *S. lavandulifolia* or possibly *S. fruticosa*. Quincy also describes a third variety, *Salvia sylvestris*, 'which is the *scorodonia* or *Salvia agrestis* of Gerhard, but is not used in the Shops altho' much recommended by ancient Writers for possessing the same virtues as Cloves'. Gerard's 'scorodonia' is wood sage (*Teucrium scorodonia*).

Quincy goes on to describe all these sages together as:

> . . . in such Esteem, as to occasion the Verse '*Cur moriatur Homo, cui Salvia crescit in Horto?*' It is undoubtedly a very good Cephalic [nerve remedy] of the detergent kind; and thereby it likewise comes under the Class of Vulneraries, Diuretics &c. It has an Austerity unto the Palate, and makes a very good Gargarism [gargle], especially if sharpen'd with a little Acid. It makes an excellent Liquor after the manner of Tea, in Fevers, and is mighty grateful and cooling with the addition of a little lemon-juice, which with the red Sage makes it of a delightful Colour. As it is both detergent and absorbent, it is a very good and common ingredient in Diet Drinks and medicinal Ales, intended for Sweetners and Cleansers of the Blood.

Richard Brook in his early nineteenth-century *Family Herbal* (written, he says, to 'combat the reading of such trash as old Culpeper') makes the same differentiation between '*Salvia major*' and sage of virtue or '*S. minor*', describing *S. minor* leaves as 'narrower and of a whitish-green colour', which could point to Spanish sage, *S. lavandulifolia*, rather than the Greek variety which Culpeper had previously recorded under this name. Of '*S. major*' he says:

> The leaves and tops of this useful plant are used and they are best fresh; the common way of taking them in infusion, or in form of what is called sage tea, is better than any other; they are cordial, and good against all diseases of the nerves; they promote perspiration, and throw any thing out which ought to appear upon the skin. The juice of sage works by urine and promotes the menses.

He is less enthusiastic about 'sage of virtue': 'the green tops are used, and their virtues are much the same with those of the former, but they are less. It got into use from an opinion that the other was too hot, but this was idle.'

Brook's comments about sage encouraging perspiration is confusing since the plant is now recognised as an antihidrotic and will actually reduce sweating.

Many other uses have been recorded for sage over the centuries: Pliny tells us that 'a traveller who has *artemisia* and *elelisphacus* tied on him does not, they say, feel any fatigue'. The various *Tacuinum Sanitatis* of the Middle Ages (Arano, 1976) give its prime virtue as 'good for paralysis and for the nerves'—although rather confusingly these books also suggest, in direct contrast to Dioscorides, that the greatest 'danger' of sage is that it will 'remove the dark colour from the hair', a problem which can be overcome, they declare, with a rinse made from myrtle and garden crocus.

Sage was also considered a cure for plague and was an important ingredient in 'Four Thieves Vinegar', a mix originally used by grave robbers who stole from the communal burial pits of plague-ridden communities. This was made by mixing one teaspoon each of dried sage, rosemary, lavender, thyme and wormwood in 500ml (1pt) of vinegar. The robbers would take sips of the brew and soak their clothing in the mix before heading for the graveyards. It would certainly make a powerful disinfectant today, although not one for internal consumption.

A remedy for old age—and new

But while there are few significant early medical descriptions of sage as an exceptional longevity remedy, there are plenty of references in Roman and Arabic literature to its association with long and healthy living, and mediaeval elixirs for eternal life frequently included large quantities of sage, declaring that 'the desire of sage is to render man immortal' (Palaiseul, 1973). The physicians of tenth-century Salerno considered that the 'supertonic effects' of sage were only limited by death itself (Holmes, 1989).

The Romans also believed that, as well as saving life, sage could help create it, and in those days the plant was a popular infertility remedy. Women would drink sage juice for four days while abstaining from sexual intercourse. After a break of a further four days sexual relations could resume and conception was assured. William Turner (1562) relates a tale from Agrippa describing the tradition:

> if a woman drink a pound of the juice of it with a little salt, at a certain time which Physicians can tell, if she do lie with her husband, undoubtedly she shall conceive. They say when the pestilence was in a place of Egypt called Coptos, that they that remained alive after the pestilence compelled their wives to drink much of this juice, and so they had in a short time great increase of children.

Even today in many parts of Europe sage continues to be regarded as an all-purpose health-giving remedy: eating sage leaves remains popular in Italy—as the extensive use of the herb in Italian cooking well testifies—while fresh sage with bread and butter was still popular in Britain in the 1930s, according to Mrs Grieve (1931). She recounts the story of George Whitfield who lived in Oxford in the 1730s and 'lived wholesomely if sparingly on a diet of sage tea, sugar and coarse bread'. She also records that use of sage wines, teas and ales, often in combination with other herbs, remained popular in country districts. One favourite brew used equal amounts of speedwell (*Veronica officinalis*), sage and wood betony (*Stachys officinalis*), not unlike Gerard (1597) who used a similar mixture for sage ale: 'No man needeth to doubt of the wholesomnesse of sage ale being brewed as it should be with sage, scabious, betonie, spikenard, squinanth and fennell seedes'.

Gerard refers elsewhere to squinanth as a type of rush, although 'squinancy berries' was also a country name for blackcurrants, while spikenard (*Nardostachys grandiflorum*) is an Indian herb highly prized throughout the mediaeval period as an exotic and potent remedy.

All sorts of folklore

Folk tradition has it that if the sage bush thrives in a garden then so will the prosperity of the household; but if the bush withers, then business will be bad. As with other herbs which have a strong tradition of use in gynaecology or obstetrics, sage is also associated with the female members of the house. Mrs Grieve relates a Buckinghamshire belief that where sage plants flourish the 'mistress is the master' and a strong woman rules the home. Country husbands would reputedly cut down the family sage bush at night rather than have the neighbours think they were not master in their own houses.

There are also a number of European traditions associating sage with grief: Mrs Grieve tells us that it is drunk in the Jura to ease the mental anguish of grief, while Samuel Pepys records that: 'Between Gosport and Southampton we observed a little churchyard where it was customary to sow all the graves with Sage'. It is not clear whether Pepys is referring to common sage or the native English wild clary (*S. verbenaca*) which was also often found growing in old country churchyards.

Dr Frederick Arnold (in *The Flora of Sussex*, 1887) suggests that this was the result of a mediaeval practice of sowing the plant on graves in the belief that it conferred immortality; a tradition, he argued, derived from the proverb 'Why should a man die who grows sage in his garden?'—which is an interesting if rather unusual interpretation (quoted in Mabey, 1996).

CHAPTER 4

Sage Under the Microscope

A guarantee of a long and healthy life is only one of common sage's many attributes. Among its therapeutic properties which have been variously listed over the years are:

- antibacterial
- antibiotic
- antihidrotic (reduces production of body fluids)
- anti-inflammatory
- antiseptic
- antispasmodic
- antiviral
- astringent
- bile stimulant
- carminative
- circulatory stimulant
- digestive
- hypoglycaemic (reduces blood sugar levels)
- memory strengthener
- mild diuretic
- oestrogenic
- peripheral vasodilator (relaxes peripheral blood vessels)
- reduces salivation
- reduces sweating
- reduces lactation
- tonic
- uterine stimulant

Sadly, few of these actions have been verified by modern scientific testing and the official ESCOP Monograph (1996) on sage—the latest melding of agreed activities by a pan-European scientific committee—gives only two therapeutic indications:

1 For 'inflammations and infections of the mouth and throat, such as stomatitis, gingivitis and pharyngitis', largely based on the recommendations from German herbalists (Weiss, 1991; Brieskorn, 1991).
2 For 'hyperhidrosis' (excessive sweating), a recommendation

again derived from German research (Weiss, 1991; Wichtl, 1989; Rösing, 1989).

The ESCOP Monographs are aimed largely at producers of over-the-counter herbal remedies and the agreed activities they cite are likely, eventually, to be what suppliers can claim for their potions without the need for further authentication. These Monographs attempt to reflect some agreement in the different traditional uses of various herbs across Europe, so it is not surprising that a 'lowest common denominator' approach prevails and one is given only the simplest and most indisputable of therapeutic actions.

What the ESCOP Monograph fails to mention is a number of studies in recent years which have sought to verify the status of sage in folk medicine as a longevity remedy. Although limited, these studies have suggested that the plant may be an effective treatment for Alzheimer's disease, and it certainly has hormonal activity which may even put it in the 'natural hormone replacement' category.

A REMEDY FOR OLD AGE?

In 1995 researchers at the Medical Research Council's Neurochemical Pathology Unit at Newcastle General Hospital studied fifteen herbs traditionally associated with improving the memory, to see if any could be of use in halting the progressive deterioration of memory which is a main symptom of Alzheimer's disease.

The team, led by Elaine Perry (Itzhaki, 1995), set out to test whether these herbs might inhibit the action of the enzyme acetyl-cholinesterase (AChE). This enzyme acts in the body to break down acetylcholine.

Acetylcholine is one of the body's chemical messengers which transmits impulses from one nerve to another, particularly in the parasympathetic nervous system, and which also has an important message-carrying role within the brain itself. A deficiency of acetylcholine is a characteristic of Alzheimer's disease, so remedies that can combat the breakdown of this important chemical, by inhibiting the enzyme that destroys it, could be helpful for Alzheimer's sufferers.

43

Orthodox treatments have focused on the drugs Tancrine, Exelon and Aricept, which effectively inhibit AChE and so slow down the progress of the disease. Unfortunately they tend to have unpleasant side-effects—Tancrine, for example, can cause liver damage—so the researchers were hoping to find a safer alternative.

Of the fifteen plants studied in the Newcastle laboratory tests, sage extracts proved to be the most promising at inhibiting AChE. Later studies have investigated both common sage and Spanish sage oils (see review, *Herbs for Health*, 1998) and confirmed the Newcastle findings with regard to AChE.

However, as always with such studies, the aim is to isolate a single active constituent which may be responsible for the activity. Research work is expensive and there has to be a profitable drug on the horizon to justify the investment. By extracting and syn-thesising whatever it is in sage that inhibits AChE, researchers would hope to create a patentable drug for future use. Simply finding that sage has this effect is not enough—after all, anyone might grow sage and use it in this way and how would the pharma-ceutical companies gain any profits?

Work has continued at King's College Pharmacognosy Depart-ment, London (Alzheimer's Disease Society News, 1997), attempting to identify likely chemicals, and a clinical trial using sage has been planned with Alzheimer's patients by the Institute for the Health of the Elderly in Newcastle. The research is sup-ported by Shire Pharmaceuticals and progress—as always—is slow. For the best part of a decade Shire Pharmaceuticals has been working on an extract from snowdrop and daffodil bulbs (galantamine) which also inhibits AChE; by August 1998 clinical trials had demonstrated its activity in slowing deterioration among Alzheimer's patients: after a year of taking galantamine, the intel-lect of Alzheimer's patients was the same as it was when they started the trial, while those on a placebo had continued to deterio-rate significantly. A commercial product, branded as Reminyl, has finally started to be marketed in some countries.

Galantamine has taken years to reach this final commercial stage. On a similar timetable, sage extracts may become commercial as a relief for Alzheimer's within three to five years. If so, their use in Alzheimer's would come as no surprise to earlier herbalists. As John Gerard wrote in 1597:

> Sage is singular good for the head and braine, quickneth the senses and memorie, strengtheneth the sinews, restoreth health to those that have a palsie upon a moist cause, taketh away shaking and trembling of the members, and being put up into the nostrils, it draweth thin flegme out of the head.

Antioxidants are also believed to be important in treating Alzheimer's as the characteristic destruction of brain cells it involves is linked to excessive oxidation. Numerous studies in recent years have examined the antioxidant properties of various herbs—and once again, sage shows significant levels of activity.

One review of 78 common herbs (Nakatani, 1994) found that 32 demonstrated some degree of antioxidant activity when tested in lard, with rosemary (*Rosmarinus officinalis*) and sage heading the list as 'remarkably effective'. Other culinary herbs—origano (*Origanum heracleoticum*), thyme (*Thymus vulgaris*), nutmeg (*Myristica fragrans*) and turmeric (*Curcuma longa*)—were next on the list.

A Slovakian study (Takácsova *et al.*, 1995), which examined how alcoholic extracts of thyme, sage, juniper and oregano could prevent oxidation and decay of a sample of low oxidant, erucic acid-free rape seed oil, again showed that sage was the most effective of the four. A third study, this time at King's College London (Halliwell *et al.*, 1995), came up with a similar series (rosemary, sage, thyme, oregano, ginger, turmeric, cayenne and bay).

Antioxidants can be quite specific in helping different types of tissues. Cigarette smoke, for example, causes excessive oxidation of lipids in blood, so increasing the risk of heart disease. A specific to combat this particular damage is vitamin C, which also has significant antioxidant activity. Vitamin C, however, has little effect on the damage cigarette smoke does to body proteins. Other antioxidants work by scavenging free radicals which are breakdown products, produced normally in the body, that can lead to oxidation of cells; the antioxidants inactivating the free radicals by binding the offending particles to themselves.

Among common antioxidant herbs so far investigated, ginkgo is known to reduce oxidation of the cells in blood vessel walls, so making them more flexible to combat hardening of the arteries. Milk thistle (*Silybum marianum*) has a similar effect on liver cells, helping to protect against oxidising toxins.

Much of this work on antioxidants has been financed by the food industry and is aimed at producing safer, natural preservatives as an alternative to such chemicals as butylated hydroxytoluene and butylated hydroxyanisole: rosmarinic acid—found in both sage and rosemary (see below)—is eight times more antioxidant than these synthetic products.

Research on how sage affects body cells is limited, but importantly, the antioxidant properties of the plant have been associated with its non-volatile parts rather than the essential oil (Svoboda and Deans, 1990). As the oil is highly toxic (see chapter 6) this is an important finding since sage leaf infusions are perfectly safe to drink regularly. The various experiments have involved use of various organic solvents, which has made it difficult to identify just which chemicals within sage may be responsible for the antioxidant activity—it may even be a group of compounds with significant seasonal variation. After all, as we have seen, John Hill back in the 1760s (chapter 1) found that a 33 per cent alcoholic extract of the flowering tops, gathered in July when the flowers first began to open, was the most effective extract he obtained, and such precision might well be a fruitful source for future study.

Early writers like John Gerard also suggested that sage could be helpful for the 'trembling of the members'. While again there is little research to suggest that it might be of help in such 'trembling' disorders as Parkinson's disease, it is used in this condition to give symptomatic relief from the characteristic excessive salivation which can be so uncomfortable for sufferers.

Sage is not only antihidrotic, reducing excessive sweating, but tends to dry up other body fluids as well—hence its use in reducing saliva. It is obviously not as dramatic as potent extracts like atropine (from deadly nightshade, *Atropa belladonna*) also used in this way, but is an effective, gentle remedy.

Help for hormones

As well as action in reducing AChE activity and as an antioxidant, sage finds a third role in the 'third age' as a menopausal remedy. Traditionally it has been recommended for symptomatic relief of hot flushes and night sweats thanks, in part, to its antihidrotic action. It is now known that the plant also has hormonal activity so may act as an oestrogen regulator—almost as a sort of weak hormone replacement treatment.

Many familiar foodstuffs, as well as herbs, contain oestrogenic substances, often in very variable amounts, and the reasons for their presence are only beginning to be appreciated. Australian herbalist Nancy Beckham (1995) recounts a delightful story of how, in the US desert, plants produce large amounts of oestrogen in dry weather. These plants provide the quail, which live in the desert, with food, and in a dry year the high oestrogen levels act as a natural contraceptive and reduce the quail's egg-laying ability. In wet years, when food is plentiful and young quail have a much better chance of survival, the same plants have very low oestrogen levels.

At least 29 different sorts of plant oestrogens have been identified and found in more than 300 different foods or herbs, and these may take the form of coumestrols, isoflavones, lignans and other plant sterols (table 1). Research on plant sterols is limited, with most work focusing on β-sitosterol which has an oestrogen-like action in humans: β-sitosterols in pumpkin seeds and saw palmetto berries (*Serenoa repens*), for example, are believed to be responsible for combating benign prostate enlargement in men.

Table 1: Some plant sources for oestrogenically active compounds (Beckham, 1995)

COUMESTROL	ISOFLAVONES	ZEARALENONE	OESTROGENS	LIGNANS	OTHERS
Soya sprouts	Soya beans	Corn	Liquorice	Linseed	Sage
Alfalfa	Alfalfa	Oats	French beans	Rye	Fennel
Red clover	Parsley	Barley	Apples	Buckwheat	Celery
Green beans	Chickpeas	Rye	Rice	Millet	Black cohosh
Red beans	Whole grains	Wheat		Oilseeds	Corn oil
Split peas	Cherries	Rice		Sesame seeds	Alcoholic drinks
Olives		Peas		Sunflower seed	Carrots
		Sesame		Dried seaweed	Cabbage
		Amaranth		Legumes	Broccoli
				Whole grains	Rhubarb
					Potato
					Squash
					Peas
					Hops
					Aniseed
					Dang Gui
					Linseed
					Olive oil
					Sunflower
					Garlic
					Beetroot
					Plum
					Pumpkin
					Marrow
					Baker's yeast

The 'oestrogenic principle' in sage has not been fully categorised, although some studies suggest that it is related to the toxic chemical thujone which is concentrated in the essential oil (Chevallier, 1996). Thujone is found in greater concentrations in *S. officinalis* than in Greek or Spanish sage. However, both these varieties have similar reputations as gynaecological remedies—Culpeper, for example, identifies 'sage of virtue' (probably *S. fruticosa*) as a menstrual stimulant, while nineteenth-century herbal writers like Richard Brook suggest that sage and 'sage of virtue' have virtually identical actions. If thujone was solely responsible for the oestrogenic activity then this sort of comparison seems unlikely. Similarly, as already noted, commercial supplies of sage are often heavily adulterated with Greek sage (*S. fruticosa*). This has a much greater 1,8-cineole content (Svoboda and Deans, 1990) and also a far lower thujone content than *S. officinalis*. If thujone

48

is largely responsible for sage's oestrogenic content this would obviously be significant for anyone hoping to use the herb as a hormonal remedy. However, commercial sage is used perfectly adequately for a wide range of menopausal problems so clearly other, more important, constituents are involved.

Nancy Beckham recommends that her menopausal patients eat two cups a day of vegetables known to be high in oestrogen—in the form of sprouted seeds, soya beans, legumes or whole grains—while supplementing these with high-oestrogen herbs like sage and fennel. She maintains that it is extremely unlikely that high levels of plant oestrogens will increase the risk of cancer, as is suggested with hormone replacement therapy. Calculated in 'diethyl stilboestrol equivalents'—a potent synthetic oestrogen—the typical daily intake from the contraceptive pill is rated at 2500µg, menopausal hormone replacement treatment at 500–1000µg daily, 20g (¾oz) of dried soya bean sprouts (70 ppm of coumesterol) at 0.5µg, and 100g (4oz) of French beans (containing 6 ppm of oestrodiol) at 0.09µg. These natural amounts may seem tiny—but often all the body needs is tiny amounts of hormone to readjust the natural balance, rather than the megadoses of modern medicine.

OTHER ATTRIBUTES

Over the years several of sage's other properties have been confirmed in studies. It is recognised as very effective at reducing sweating, and its long tradition as a remedy for mouth and gum problems has been confirmed in trials which showed that it can reduce dental plaque, has antiviral activity against the virus causing mouth ulcers, and will reduce gum inflammations (some of these are discussed in more detail in chapter 5).

Like other culinary herbs, sage is both strongly flavoured and strongly antimicrobial: one recent study (Sharman and Billing, 1998) maintains that humans have developed their taste for many culinary herbs and spices largely because these plants tend to be so effective at killing bacteria. 'Traits that are beneficial are transmitted culturally and genetically,' says Professor Paul Sharman, 'and that includes the taste receptors in our mouths. People who enjoyed food with antibacterial spices probably were healthier, especially in hot climates. They lived longer and left more offspring. The ultimate reason for using spices is to kill food-borne bacterial and fungi.'

Culinary flavourings like thyme, cumin and tarragon will kill up to 80 per cent of bacteria, and sage is not far below this level. 'Everything we do with food—drying, cooking, smoking, salting or adding spices—is an attempt to keep from being poisoned by our microscopic competitors,' says Professor Sharman. 'They're constantly mutating and evolving to stay ahead of us. One way we reduce food-borne illnesses is to add another spice to the recipe.'

All the more reason to eat plenty of sage.

ALL SORTS OF CONSTITUENTS

As with many herbs, the active constituents in sage have not been fully identified or categorised. The plant contains an impressive cocktail of chemicals, although which are responsible for its various activities is still largely unknown. Among those that have been identified are:

- an assortment of monoterpenoids, sesquiterpenoids and other substances found in the volatile oil, including: 1,8-cineole, caryophyllene, linalol, borneol, camphor, carysalvene, α-pinene, linalyl acetate, and many other terpenes (Müller *et al.*, 1992; Brieskorn and Dalferth, 1964; Jalsenjak *et al.*, 1987); key constituents of the oil are α- and β-thujones at concentrations of up to 60 per cent and 10 per cent respectively (Steinegger and Hänsel, 1992), although concentrations of all these substances can vary significantly between different specimens (Svoboda and Deans, 1990)
- monoterpene glycosides (Croteau *et al.*, 1984; van der Dries and Baerheim Svendsen, 1989)
- bitter diterpenes such as picrosalvin or carnosol, carnosolic acid and derivatives like carnisol (Wagner

et al., 1984; Rutherford *et al.*, 1992; Brieskorn and Dömling, 1969)

- triterpenoids including oleanic acid, ursolic acid and derivatives (Brieskorn, 1991; Brieskorn and Kapadia, 1980)
- flavonoids, including genkwanin, 6-methoxygenkwanin, hispidulin, luteolin, salvigenin, 5-methoxysalvigenin (Brieskorn and Biechele, 1971; Brieskorn and Kapadia, 1979)
- phenolic compounds including caffeic, chlorogenic, ellagic, ferulic, gallic and rosmarinic acid (Gracza and Ruff, 1984; Wagner *et al.*, 1984; Petri *et al.*, 1988),
- oestrogenic substances
- tannins (3–8 per cent)—notably salviatannin, a condensed catechin (Murko *et al.*, 1974)
- resin

Finding explanations

The actions of these various chemicals help to explain sage's properties, although many are not fully understood. Monoterpenes and sesquiterpenes, for example, are usually strongly antimicrobial and can also have a carminative effect (this is especially true of thujone). Studies have also suggested that thujone is active against bacteria like *Escherichia coli*, *Shigella sonnei*, *Salmonella* spp. *Klebsella ozanae*, *Bacillus subtilis* and such fungi as *Candida albicans*, *C. krusie*, *C. pseudotropicalis*, *Torulopsis globrata*, and *Cryptococcus neoformans* (Newall *et al.*, 1996). One research study proposed that pinene was responsible for antispasmodic activity (Taddei *et al.*, 1988).

The diterpenes, found in the leafy parts of the plant rather than the oil, show antiviral activity specifically against the virus responsible for mouth ulcers or aphthous stomatitis (Chiba *et al.*, 1992).

Phenols tend also to be antiseptic, while rosmarinic acid is highly antioxidant and anti-inflammatory. Studies suggest that rosmarinic acid is active at reducing dental plaque and gum inflammations (van Dyke *et al.*, 1986)—which helps explain why sage has been used in tooth powders and pastes since the Middle Ages.

Useful nutrients

Sage supplies more than just potent chemicals with each cup of infusion. A study by American herbalist James Duke (1997) analysed the mineral content of a cup of sage tea based on one teaspoon of dried herb in a cup of boiled water (table 2). Obviously this is going to be very variable, depending on where the sage was grown and the time of year when it was harvested, but it provides a useful indication of sage's many hidden and beneficial talents.

Table 2: Sage tea

MINERAL	MG	%RDA[*]
Iron	17.6	117
Magnesium	428.0	107
Calcium	620	62
Potassium	2006	50
Zinc	4	27
Sodium	18	<1

[*]recommended daily allowance

Duke suggests that to obtain the highest extraction rate for minerals like these it is best to make enough for three cups and leave the tea to infuse overnight. In the morning strain the mixture and reheat enough for each cup as required.

CHAPTER 5

Using Sage in Home Remedies

Although sage's many therapeutic properties have not all been thoroughly investigated or officially recognised, the herb still remains one of our most effective household remedies for a wide range of ills. A shrubby common sage bush (see chapter 8) will remain green through the year, and while the quality of the leaves will vary with the changing seasons, they will still be available to pick fresh at almost any time. Alternatively, they can be gathered and dried to provide a store for the winter.

HARVESTING AND DRYING

The leaves are most aromatic and strongest during May or just before flowering in July. Choose a dry, sunny day after any morning dew has cleared; clip the bush to collect stems of leaves and flowering racemes and tie them in small bunches of four or five sprigs.

All herbs need to be dried as quickly as possible, and away from bright sunlight to preserve the aromatic ingredients and prevent oxidation of other chemicals. An airing cupboard, spare room, dry garden shed or barn are ideal, but avoid hanging herbs in the garage as they can easily absorb petrol fumes and will be unusable. A good circulation of air is essential: professional growers often keep a low-powered fan heater running. Ideally the temperature in the drying room should be between 20–32°C/70–90°F and should never go above 38°C/100°F.

In warm conditions the sage will be completely dry within five or six days, sometimes even less. The longer the plant takes to dry, the more likely it is to discolour and lose its flavour. When dry, the leaves and flowering tops can be easily stripped from the stems, crumbled gently, and stored in clean dry jars or pots with an airtight lid. If the herbs are stored when still slightly damp they will go mouldy. Jars should ideally be of coloured glass or pottery, or kept out of direct sunlight which speeds deterioration. Do not store herbs in metal or plastic containers.

Label the jar with details of the variety, source and date. If dried and stored properly, sage will keep for at least 12–18 months without significant deterioration. Too many cooks keep a jar of sage at the back of the kitchen cupboard for years, ready for the annual turkey stuffing at Christmas: it might be acceptable for some dishes but will certainly have lost many of its active constituents over the years and be far from ideal as a medicine.

Some people use a microwave oven for drying herbs, but researchers at the West of Scotland College in Auchincruive found some years ago that microwaving aromatic herbs actually led to changes in their chemical composition as the radiation transformed the reactive molecules in the plant oils. They found that entirely new substances, of unknown toxicity or efficacy, were produced. It therefore seems best to avoid this technique for an aromatic plant like sage.

BUYING DRIED HERBS

Rubbed dried sage is readily available commercially and *Dan Shen* roots can be bought from specialist Chinese herbalists, but other varieties will need to be grown and dried at home. Always buy the minimum quantity you need to avoid unnecessary storage for long periods at home (no more than 250g/½lb) and avoid buying herbs which are being displayed in shops in clear glass jars on sunny shelves and look as though they may have been there for some time. Old stock can be a problem when buying ready-dried common sage as the plant tends to look the same grey-green colour no matter how old it is. Try smelling the herb if possible to ensure a good, fresh aroma; ideally buy organically grown sage.

Try to check that the herbs supplies are actually what you want—mistakes do happen and adulteration with *S. fruticosa* is almost inevitable with commercial supplies.

Ready-made sage tincture is available from the suppliers listed at the end of this book, although in the UK it is not so easy to buy sage ointments, creams or oils. Powdered sage can also be bought in capsules. Arkopharma, for example, market 220mg of sage in capsules as Phytomenopause.

Either dried or fresh sage can be used in making simple home remedies. The herb can be used in infusions or teas, tinctures, creams, ointments, infused oils, poultices or compresses. Full details for making these different remedies are given below.

MAKING HOME-MADE REMEDIES

Infusions

An infusion is simply a tea made by steeping the herb in freshly boiled water for ten minutes. Traditionally, herbal infusions were made once a day using 15–30g (½–1oz) of dried herb to 500ml (1pt) of boiled water. This is sufficient for three wine-glass doses.

Dried sage is, however, a bulky, light herb and also very potent—25g (1oz) of sage would be the equivalent of about ten very slightly rounded tablespoons, which is far more than is necessary or desirable. A better guide for sage is a maximum of 5g (¼oz) per 500ml (1pt) of water, which is roughly the equivalent of 2 very slightly rounded tablespoonfuls. Alternatively, for a single dose use 3 level or 1 heaped teaspoon.

To make the infusion, pour freshly boiled water over the sage and infuse for ten minutes, before straining and drinking the mix. A tisane cup (which has an inner ceramic pot with a strainer at the bottom) is ideal to use for making single doses or, if you prefer to make a single brew to last the day, put the sage into a ceramic or glass teapot or jug (with lid), and add the water. It is important for this to be just off the boil, otherwise many aromatic constituents will be lost in the excessive steam. After infusing for about 10– 15 minutes, strain through a sieve or tea strainer, as with conventional tea leaves. Sweeten with a little honey according to taste. The strained infusion can be reheated before each dose if preferred.

It is best to make enough infusion for only one day's doses, although any surplus can be stored in a refrigerator for up to 48 hours. If using fresh herb you need three times as much to allow for the additional weight of water in fresh plant material.

These same infusions can be used as a mouthwash or gargle for throat and gum problems. The ESCOP Monograph on sage (see chapter 4), suggests a maximum of 3g of sage per cup for gargles and mouthwashes and 1–1.5g per cup for the infusion. These sorts of doses are also likely to be recommended on therapeutic sage products sold commercially.

Tinctures

A tincture is an alcoholic extraction of the active constituents of a herb made by soaking the dried or fresh plant material in a mixture of alcohol and water for two weeks and then straining the mix through a wine press or jelly bag.

Although any alcohol can be used to make tinctures, not all are safe to drink so great care needs to be taken with home production. Commercially produced tinctures are usually made from 95 per cent ethyl alcohol diluted to the required strength with water. Methyl alcohol is extremely poisonous and must never be taken internally, and although some recommend isopropyl alcohol (rubbing alcohol) for tincture-making, this is also very toxic and should be avoided. A more complex alcohol is glycerol or glycerine (propan-1,2,3-triol, available from chemists) which can be used and has the benefit of being very low cost, but the resulting tinctures are slightly slimy to the taste.

In many European countries the supply of high-grade alcohol is strictly controlled by state customs and excise departments, which can make home-made tincture production more complicated. A few are more flexible: in France, for example, it is possible to buy high strength, inexpensive ethyl alcohol mixtures (around 45 per cent or more) which are sold in supermarkets for bottling fruit, but in Britain and elsewhere the easiest way to obtain suitable alcohol for tincture-making is to buy a basic quality vodka.

Commercial sage tincture is usually made with a 45 per cent alcohol/water mixture [45ml (1½fl oz) of alcohol and 55ml (2fl oz) of water per 100ml (3½fl oz) of mixture]. This can be difficult to replicate at home as vodka and other commercially available spirits are usually 37.5 per cent alcohol. However, since John Hill (chapter 1) favoured a 33 per cent mixture, this would no doubt be just as good for home use—especially if gathering your herb in July as he suggested.

A 33 per cent alcohol/water mix has 33cl (11½fl oz) of alcohol and 67cl (23½fl oz) of water per litre (35fl oz), while standard vodka is 37.5cl (13fl oz) of alcohol and 62.5cl (22fl oz) of water per litre (35fl oz). To make this into a 33 per cent mix you simply need to add an additional 100ml (3½fl oz) of water to your 1 litre (35fl oz) of vodka.

Standard tinctures are usually made in the weight:volume proportion 1:5 (i.e. 1kg of herb to 5 litres of alcohol/water mixture or 1lb of herb to 5pt of liquid). For home use mixing 100g (4oz) of herb with ½ litre (25fl oz) of the diluted vodka mixture is usually a sufficient quantity to make at any one time. If using fresh herb then, as with infusions, you need three times as much because of the water content in the leaves.

To make sage tincture, simply put the required quantity of herb into a large jar (ideally an old-fashioned glass screw-top sweet jar). Then cover with the vodka/water mixture and store in a cool place for two weeks, shaking the jar occasionally. Strain the mixture through a wine press or jelly bag and then store the tincture in clean, dark glass bottles. Tinctures will general last for two years or more without deterioration.

Normal maximum recommended dose for sage tincture is 4ml (80 drops) a day taken in 3–4 doses of 20–25 drops.

Ointments and creams

Ointments contain only oils or fats and will form a separate protective layer over the skin, so they are ideal where the skin is already weak or soft or where some protection is needed from additional moisture. Traditionally, ointments were made using animal fats and the simplest method is to heat dried sage in melted lard or Vaseline for a couple of hours.

Melt 100g (4oz) of Vaseline over a low heat and then add 25g (1oz) of dried sage. Continue heating until the herb feels crisp and crunchy and then pour through a fine sieve or jelly bag directly into clean, sterilised glass jars. Pre-heat the glass jars in an oven (150°C/300°F/gas mark 2) for five minutes before transferring to a wire cooling rack, ready for pouring in the ointment. It will help to sterilise them and reduce the risk of cracking the glass when the hot ointment is added.

Creams are made from a mixture of oils or fats and water which are miscible with the skin (they mix in with or can be absorbed by it). They can easily be made at home using emulsifying ointment (available from pharmacists). This is a mixture of oils (usually hydrocarbons or paraffins) which can be blended with a certain proportion of water to make a cream. The usual method involves melting the emulsifying ointment in a double saucepan or *bain marie*, then adding the dried herb and water (or a water/alcohol mixture) and simmering for 2–3 hours. Typical proportions with this method would be: 300g (11oz) emulsifying ointment, 135ml (5fl oz) glycerol, 165ml (6fl oz) water and 60g (2¼ oz) dried sage.

A natural alternative to emulsifying ointment is to use:

> 100ml (4fl oz) sunflower oil (or similar)
> 25g (1oz) white beeswax
> 25g (1oz) anhydrous lanolin
> 75ml (3fl oz) water
> 25ml (1fl oz) glycerol
> 50g (2oz) dried sage

In this case melt the solid fats (as with emulsifying ointment) and then add the other ingredients.

After simmering the mixture, press it through a fine nylon sieve, jelly bag or wine press and then stir constantly until it is cool to prevent the oils and water from reseparating. If this happens, add a little more emulsifying ointment or beeswax and re-heat for a little longer. Finally, store the cream in clean, airtight plastic or glass jars.

Home-made sage cream will usually keep for several months and is best stored in a cool larder or refrigerator.

Infused oils

Infused sage oil can be used instead of the ointment and also makes a suitable massage oil for aromatherapy (see chapter 6). There are two techniques: hot infusion or cold infusion. The hot method is ideal for the older sage leaves at any time of year, while the cold is nice to use in the summer with sage flowers, flowering tops or young shoots.

Hot infusion: Heat 100g (4oz) of dried [300g (12oz) fresh] sage in 500ml (1pt) of sunflower oil (or similar) in a double saucepan over water for about three hours. Remember to refill the lower saucepan with hot water from time to time to prevent it from boiling dry. After about three hours the oil will take on a greenish colour. Strain the mix through a sieve, muslin bag or wine press and store in clean glass bottles, away from direct sunlight.

Cold infusion: Because the oil is not heated in this method, you can use good quality seed oils that are rich in essential fatty acids (EFA)— such as *gamma*-linolenic or *cis*-linoleic—which have significant therapeutic properties. Oils high in EFA include walnut, safflower and pumpkin oils. Fill a large, clear glass jar with sage racemes and flowers and cover completely with oil. This is important as any herb exposed to the air may go mouldy and the mixture will be spoilt. Leave the jar on a sunny windowsill or in the greenhouse for at least three weeks and then strain and store the mixture as with hot oils.

Poultices and compresses

Compresses are used to accelerate healing of wounds or muscle injuries. They are basically cloth pads soaked in herbal extracts and usually applied hot to painful limbs, swellings or strains. Use a clean piece of cotton, cotton wool, linen or surgical gauze soaked in a hot, strained infusion, decoction or tincture (diluted with hot water) and apply to the affected area. When the compress cools repeat using fresh, hot mixture.

Poultices have a very similar action to compresses but involve applying the whole herb to an affected area directly, rather than using a liquid extract. Poultices are usually applied hot for swellings, sprains or to draw pus. Renew the hot poultice as it cools or place a hot-water bottle on top to keep it hot.

To make a poultice, simply bruise fresh sage leaves or mix in a food processor for a few seconds, then spread the mixture onto gauze and apply to the affected area. Dried sage leaves or sage powder need mixing with hot water to make a soft paste, then squeeze out any surplus liquid and spread the residue on gauze or apply directly to the area affected.

If putting a poultice directly to the skin, apply a little vegetable oil first to prevent it from sticking.

SAGE AND SIMPLE AILMENTS

The easiest way to use sage at home is as an infusion. However, in the remedies given below it is generally just as effective to use tincture instead. Where a 'standard infusion' is suggested, see the section on making infusions on p. 55 for recommended quantities. An equivalent dose of tincture will be 20–25 drops.

CAUTIONS: sage should be avoided in pregnancy, and by those who have epilepsy or high blood pressure.

ANXIETY, DEPRESSION AND NERVOUS STRESS
Many herbalists consider sage to be a restoring tonic herb which helps to calm and stimulate the nervous system. The infusion is recommended in parts of Europe for a wide range of nervous disorders, dizziness (vertigo) and depression (Schauenberg and Paris, 1974). The French phytotherapist Jean Valnet recommends a 'stimulating wine' made by steeping 80g (1½oz) of sage leaves in a litre (1pt) of red or white wine for a week. This should then be taken in doses of 1–3 tablespoons after meals.

USING SAGE IN HOME REMEDIES

ASTHMA

Sage has a long tradition of treating chronic coughs—it was once regularly used for consumption (tuberculosis) and for severe coughs with blood-tinged phlegm. Such ailments need professional help, but sage can still be useful for less severe problems.

In asthma the small bronchial tubes in the lungs tighten, making it difficult for the sufferer to breathe out and leading to the characteristic wheeze. The tubes also fill with a sticky mucus instead of the usual lubricating fluid phlegm. Herbal smoking mixtures are a traditional remedy and sage is still available in commercially made herbal cigarettes as an asthma remedy. These can be made at home by rolling a mixture of dried sage, dried red clover flowers (*Trifolium pratense*) and crushed anise or fennel seeds in conventional cigarette papers.

Alternatively try tightly rolling crushed sage into a cigar-shaped roll using 2–3 layers of tissue paper. Cut this into 2.5cm (1in) slices (rather like moxa sticks used in Chinese moxibustion treatments), then put the slice on a saucer or tin lid, place on a heat-proof surface and light the top. It should smoulder happily for 10–15 minutes while you can inhale the fumes.

POOR APPETITE

Like many bitter-tasting herbs, sage can be used as an appetite stimulant. Its tonic action would also help where lack of appetite is associated with debility and convalescence. Use 1 level teaspoon of dried sage or 3–4 fresh leaves to a cup of water as an infusion and drink about 30 minutes before meals to stimulate the digestion and appetite.

BREAST-FEEDING

Sage's combined antihidrotic and oestrogenic properties make it ideal for drying breast milk—either at weaning or if there is an excess when breast-feeding. To reduce milk flow take one cup of sage tea (½–1 teaspoon of dried herb per cup) at night and repeat at mid-day if the flow remains excessive. At weaning make a standard infusion and drink three cups of sage tea during the day.

Continue until milk flow reduces significantly, while discouraging any of baby's attempts to suck.

As a warm, dry herb sage was viewed by earlier Galenic physicians (see chapter 3) as a remedy for cold, damp conditions, including thin, watery nasal catarrh. Sage is worth adding to catarrhal remedies used for colds, influenza or allergic rhinitis. It is also worth remembering all those recommendations from early authors that sage is good for 'watery' or 'thin phlegm', so do not use the herb for the sort of thick nasal congestion which can characterise sinusitis or some feverish colds.

Combine equal amounts of dried sage and peppermint (or spearmint if you find peppermint too heating or are making the remedy for young children, who should always avoid peppermint as it can irritate the digestive system) and use 1 heaped teaspoon per cup as a warming brew for chills and watery catarrh.

The same mix can also be used as a steam inhalation: pour 500ml (1pt) of boiling water over 1 tablespoon of the mixture in a basin; lean over the basin and cover both it and your head with a towel while inhaling the steam for as long as you can bear it.

COUGHS

Although little used as a cough remedy today, sage was once a popular choice for chronic respiratory problems such as chronic bronchitis. It is best used in combination with more active expectorants, such as elecampane root (*Inula helenium*), marshmallow leaf (*Althaea officinalis*) and white horehound (*Marrubium vulgare*). Syrups are especially soothing for coughs, and a supply of sage syrup produced from the flowering tops of the plant in July is a useful household standby both for sore throats and to add to other cough mixtures (add 1 teaspoon of syrup per dose).

To make a syrup, brew a strong infusion of sage (2 tablespoons of herb to 500ml (1pt) of boiling water and strain well). Put the strained infusion in a stainless steel or ceramic saucepan and add 500g (1lb) of unrefined sugar or honey. Heat and stir constantly while the sugar or honey dissolves and then simmer until you have a thin syrup, stirring all the time. Store the syrup in clean glass bottles stoppered with a cork: syrups tend to ferment and a tightly screwed stopper may cause the bottle to explode.

CRAMP AND PAIN

As a warming herb, sage baths were once a popular remedy to ease stiff limbs and reduce cramp. Either strain a cup of strong infusion (1 tablespoon of sage with a cup of water) into the bathwater, or add this to 500ml (1pt) of hot water and use it to soak a compress which can be applied directly to the aching area. Hot poultices can be used in the same way.

John Gerard recommended wrapping red sage leaves with hot ashes splashed with vinegar in a cloth and holding this 'unto the side of those that are troubled with a grievous stitch, [it] taketh away the paine presently; the same helpeth greatly the extremitie of the pleurisie'.

A cup of hot sage infusion can also be added to a foot bath to relieve aching feet and act as a generally warming remedy for chills and cold limbs—ideal after a cold, wet winter walk!

DIARRHOEA

There are many causes of the frequent loose or liquid bowel motions of diarrhoea—from food poisoning and overeating to stress and anxiety. Sudden diarrhoea is most commonly caused by some sort of gastro-intestinal infection, especially if others who shared the same meal are similarly affected. Diarrhoea and vomiting are the body's natural reaction to an infecting organism and are often the best way of getting rid of it quickly.

Like many herbal diarrhoea remedies, sage is not intended to stop the diarrhoea—more to soothe the discomfort and help the body combat any infection. The herb is strongly antimicrobial and the tannin also makes it highly astringent to combat soreness and inflammation in the lower bowel.

Drink a cup of standard infusion every three to four hours while symptoms persist, or use 50 drops of tincture in a little warm water. Diarrhoea is very dehydrating and it is important to increase fluid intake during such bouts. This is especially important for small children.

FLATULENCE

Wind, whether it goes up or down, is usually more of an embarrassment than an indicator of serious health problems. Flatulence can be accompanied by stomach pains, bloating and cramps, with rumblings in the lower bowel adding to the embarrassment.

Diet is often to blame and some foods are intrinsically very 'windy': old herbals usually stress this point with regard to beans and brassicas, and traditional recipes added carminative herbs to reduce the problem.

Many culinary herbs, including sage, are effective carminatives which will not only enhance the flavour of our food but will also stimulate and soothe the digestive system, so reducing the risk of wind and indigestion. Use sage in cooking (see chapter 9) or drink a cup of sage tea after meals: use 1 teaspoon of dried herb or four large fresh leaves per cup.

CAUTION: Chronic flatulence may be a symptom of more serious illness; seek professional help if symptoms persist.

GUM PROBLEMS

Gum diseases, such as gingivitis and bleeding gums, are usually the result of poor oral hygiene and if untreated can lead to loosening and loss of teeth. Brushing regularly and correctly is important, as is eating foods which contain roughage and can help clean the teeth as they are chewed. Sage is an astringent and antiseptic to help combat any bacteria and tonify gum tissue. Make half the standard infusion mixture, strain well and use half the mix as a mouthwash in the morning and half before going to bed at night. Alternatively, add 1 teaspoon of sage tincture to a tumbler of water and use half of this for each mouthwash.

USING SAGE IN HOME REMEDIES

GREYING HAIR
Sage is a traditional remedy for restoring colour to greying hair. Make a standard infusion, strain well and use this as the final rinse after shampooing. Drink a daily cup of sage tea as an added energy boost.

INDIGESTION AND MINOR DIGESTIVE UPSETS
As an effective carminative (see Flatulence, p. 64), sage is useful for indigestion and weak digestion. It is also bitter, so helps to stimulate the liver and generally improve digestive function. A cup of infusion immediately after eating makes a pleasant end to the meal, or you can use equal amounts of fennel seed and sage (1–2 teaspoons of the mix per cup). Adding sage in cooking (see chapter 9) will be just as effective.

CAUTION: Chronic indigestion may be a symptom of more serious illness; seek professional help if symptoms persist.

INSECT BITES AND STINGS
For most people insect bites and stings lead to little more than local irritation which eases in a few days. Sage is an ideal home first aid remedy to ease the discomfort and can also help reduce infection in more severe bites or where allergic reaction leads to weeping dermatitis.

Simply rub fresh sage leaves onto the sting, or if it is especially sore, chop a few fresh leaves in a small food processor and apply these to the affected area as a poultice. In France, sage ointment is commercially available and is still the preferred remedy for insect bites and minor grazes in many households. Home-made sage ointments, creams or infused oils make suitable alternatives to fresh leaves.

CAUTION: for an unfortunate minority stings can lead to very severe allergic reaction (anaphylactic shock) which may prove fatal if left untreated. Typical symptoms include dizziness, sickness, breathing problems and marked swelling of the affected area. Immediate emergency medical treatment is essential in such cases.

LARYNGITIS

Laryngitis is an inflammation of the voice box or larynx and vocal cords, usually due to a viral or bacterial infection. It can cause hoarseness or even a complete loss of voice. Sage is a specific for all sorts of throat and mouth inflammations. Use a well-strained, cooled standard infusion as a mouthwash in tumbler doses as often as possible (at least every two hours, but every 30 minutes is better if you can). Alternatively use 50 drops of sage tincture in half a tumbler of warm water. Swallow the infusion rather than spitting it out after each gargle, to benefit from sage's antibacterial properties in combating the infection. In severe cases 5–10 drops of myrrh tincture (*Commiphora molmol*) or 2 drops of cayenne tincture (*Capsicum* spp.) added to the gargle can help.

A steam inhalation is also useful: either pour boiling water over a handful of fresh sage leaves or add 2 drops of Spanish sage oil to a bowl of boiling water. Lean over the basin and cover your head and the basin with a towel. Inhale deeply for as long as you can or until the water cools and the steam subsides. On cold days stay indoors in a warm room for at least half an hour after any steam inhalation.

To combat the infection you can take daily capsules of garlic or echinacea tablets (up to 600mg, three times daily) which are available from health food shops and pharmacies.

CAUTION: if symptoms persist for more than a few days then professional investigation is needed in case there is some major problem such as a growth causing the hoarseness.

LATE ONSET DIABETES

Late onset diabetes is an all too common result of a lifetime of the worst Western diets, with too many sugars and an irregular pattern of meals. Many herbs, including sage, are now known to reduce blood sugar levels, so can be used in conjunction with a carefully controlled diet to help maintain normal levels.

Elderly diabetics are usually given urine-testing kits so that they can monitor sugar levels, so doses of suitable herbal teas can be varied as necessary. In general 2 cups a day of standard sage infusion will provide the necessary regulation; increase to 3–4 cups if need be. Other useful hypoglycaemic herbs include fenugreek (*Trigonella foenum-graecum*), bilberry leaves (*Vaccinium myrtillus*), stinging nettle (*Urtica dioica*) and goat's rue (*Galega officinalis*). These can be used in combination with sage (never more than 2 teaspoons of the mixture to a single cup) to vary the flavour of your daily brew.

CAUTION: insulin-dependent diabetics need to take great care when using hypoglycaemic herbs, unless under professional guidance.

POOR MEMORY

Sage's traditional role in strengthening the memory and improving concentration in the elderly is being confirmed by modern research (see chapter 4), so taking a daily cup or two of sage as we grow older may be beneficial for all of us. Use half a teaspoon of dried sage or two fresh leaves per cup. Rosemary (*Rosmarinus officinalis*) and gotu kola (*Centella asiatica*) have a similar reputation and will combine well with sage. Make a mixture containing equal amounts of all three herbs and use 1 teaspoon per cup of infusion, 1–2 times daily.

Nicholas Culpeper (1653) suggests that a 'conserve of sage flowers' is an ideal remedy to 'help the memory, warning and quickening the senses'. If you enjoy jam-making and have flowers from home-grown sage bushes, then cover them with water in a saucepan and simmer with an equal amount of chopped lemon peel for 20–30 minutes. Add an equal volume of sugar syrup and continue cooking until the mixture is ready to set. Alternatively, follow the sage jelly recipe given on p. 111, using flowers instead of leaves.

MENOPAUSAL PROBLEMS

For most women the menopause passes by with little more inconvenience than occasional hot flushes and night sweats. Periods often stop suddenly without further problem, or else gradually fade away in an irregular pattern.

For others, the picture is quite different. It can be a time of major emotional upheaval, depression, weight gain and heavy bleeding. Today, many of these symptoms may be treated by hormone replacement therapy which boosts oestrogen levels, although critics still have doubts about the long-term effects of such treatment.

Sage has been a popular remedy for menopausal ills for generations—although we are only starting to understand its oestrogenic activity. A regular cup of standard sage infusion (up to three times a day) or 25 drops of tincture in a little water (up to three times daily) is often enough to restore balance and eliminate tiresome hot flushes and excessive sweating.

If menopausal emotional upsets are also a problem, combine sage with an equal amount of mugwort (*Artemisia vulgaris*) and lemon balm (*Melissa officinalis*) and use this in regular infusions (1 teaspoon per cup, up to three times daily).

MENSTRUAL PROBLEMS

Sage has been used for menstrual problems at least since the days of Pliny and Dioscorides (see chapter 3), although its dangerous potency as an abortifacient has been recognised for just as long (see p. 34). The herb is classified as an emmenagogue and stimulates menstrual flow due to its oestrogenic activity. It can be helpful in regulating the menstrual cycle and is valuable in cases of scanty or absent menstruation, helping to stimulate and normalise flow.

It is important to remember that menstrual activity does vary enormously, and what is quite normal for one woman would be considered very strange by another. If a limited flow lasting only a couple of days is the normal pattern, then in most cases that is fine. Sage can be helpful if this is a change from the established pattern or where irregular or weak menstruation is a symptom of an underlying hormonal problem or infertility.

As an effective antiseptic sage can also be useful for gynae-cological problems associated with infection—as in pelvic inflammatory disease, salpingitis, abnormal vaginal discharges (leucorrhoea), or trichomonas infection. Sage can be taken internally as well as being used as a vaginal douche or in creams applied directly to the vagina.

Special douching kits are available from chemists and are made up of a bag with its own tube and nozzle. Put a well-strained cup of infusion into the bag, lie on your back with legs raised and insert the tube into the vagina and allow the douche to flow over the area. A simple alternative is to use a small plastic spray bottle filled with infusion and spray the vaginal area instead.

To combat the infection, take 3 × 200mg capsules of echinacea three times a day as the prime antibiotic remedy, and support this with 20 drops each of sage and pulsatilla (*Anemone pulsatilla*) tinctures three times daily.

Sage infusion can be used on its own or combined with equal amounts of lady's mantle (*Alchemilla xanthoclora*), St John's wort (*Hypericum perforatum*), chamomile flowers (*Matricaria recutita*) or white deadnettle (*Lamium album*). Alternatively, add 2 drops of Spanish sage oil (see p. 77) to 250ml (½pt) of water in your spray bottle and use that instead.

Sage is also helpful with premenstrual syndrome which can develop late in life during the years leading up to the menopause— again this is largely due to its oestrogenic activity. Regular sage infusions or doses of tincture during the ten days before a period is due can help. Depression and emotional upsets are often associated with this sort of PMS, so combine the herb with equal amounts of motherwort (*Leonurus cardiaca*), vervain (*Verbena officinalis*) and St John's wort (*Hypericum perforatum*).

NOTE: Absence of menstruation may be due to pregnancy, so before using sage to stimulate unexpected scanty menstruation, take a pregnancy test. Absence of periods (amenorrhoea) is also associated with abnormally low body-weight and may be a sign of anorexia nervosa, excessive exercise, emotional stress, or a problem with regaining normal menstruation after coming off the oral contraceptive pill. **Professional treatment is advisable in all these cases.**

MENTAL CONFUSION IN THE ELDERLY
Mental confusion in the elderly may be associated with senile dementia and Alzheimer's disease, and sage (see chapter 4) is now known to slow down the progression of this disease significantly.

Confusion can also be linked to a hardening of the cerebral arteries which leads to a reduced blood supply to the brain, and old people become susceptible to 'drop attacks' or sudden black-outs, as well as appearing more confused and forgetful.

One of the traditional remedies for improving cerebral circulation is wood betony (*Stachys officinalis*), while over the past few years research has demonstrated that ginkgo (*Ginkgo biloba*) can also be extremely effective.

Drinking 1–2 cups of sage and betony tea (equal amounts of each, 1–2 teaspoons of the mix per cup) is an easily available and low-cost remedy for elderly pensioners, especially since both herbs will grow happily in the garden. Ginkgo supplements, widely available in capsules and tablets, are also worth taking.

As we have seen, sage also helps reduce salivation so can be helpful for symptomatic relief in Parkinson's disease.

MOUTH ULCERS

Sage mouthwashes have long been used to combat mouth ulcers (aphthous stomatitis) and studies have shown that the leaves display antiviral activity specifically against the virus responsible (Chiba *et al.*, 1992).

Use a well-strained infusion, made from 1 level desertspoon of dried sage to a cup of water, as a mouthwash, repeating the treatment three to four times daily. Swallow the mouthwash after swilling it thoroughly around the mouth rather than spitting it out, so that the sage can carry on working between doses.

PHARYNGITIS

Pharyngitis is an inflammation of the throat behind the soft palate (pharynx) which can often be associated with tonsillitis. Typical symptoms are a sore throat and discomfort when swallowing. Use the same treatment suggested for laryngitis, and seek professional help if the problem does not ease within a few days.

SORE THROATS

A sore throat can be the first sign of a developing cold or German measles, as well as a symptoms of laryngitis, pharyngitis or tonsillitis (*q.v.*). The inflammation may be caused by viral or bacterial infection, and recurrence can be associated with stress or a reduced resistance to infection. Mild cases will often clear in two or three days, with or without treatment, but the discomfort can be eased by sage gargles. Use cups of a well-strained standard infusion— ideally every 30 minutes although this level of frequency can be a problem if you are working or travelling.

Sage can be mixed with an equal amount of rosemary (*Rosmarinus officinalis*) or lady's mantle (*Alchemilla xanthoclora*) if preferred. A tiny pinch of powdered cayenne (*Capsicum* spp.) added to each dose also helps.

EXCESSIVE SWEATING

Clinical trials (Rösing, 1989) have confirmed that sage can significantly reduce excessive sweating in cases where there is no obvious cause. Although excessive sweating can be a symptom of underlying disease (as in fevers or with the chronically ill and debilitated), some people simply sweat a great deal more than average and the problem can become a major embarrassment and social irritant.

Studies have looked at the effect of both sage infusions (4.5g of dried herb daily—about ⅙oz or 2 level tablespoons) and dried extracts in tablet form (the equivalent of 2.6g daily), and at these low doses sweating was reduced by up to 50 per cent.

Drink one cup of infusion daily using 1½ teaspoons of sage per cup, or you can use powdered sage in capsules as an alternative. The dosages used in the clinical trial would be the equivalent of four of Arkopharma's sage capsules (220mg), three times daily.

TONSILLITIS

The tonsils are small packs of lymphatic tissue at the back of the throat, which help protect the body from infection. Inflammation is usually the result of local infection, while recurrent tonsillitis, common in children, can often indicate some underlying stress on the system, such as food allergy, with the immune system having to work overtime to combat the problem.

Use the same gargle suggested for laryngitis (p. 66), repeating as often as you can during the day—every 30 minutes is ideal if possible.

CAUTION: in severe cases the tonsils can become filled with pus, causing an abscess or quinsy which may need surgical treatment. Seek professional help if symptoms worsen or do not clear within a few days.

TOOTH CARE

Sage has been a popular ingredient of herbal tooth powders and pastes for centuries. One early recipe is from *The Herbal Remedies of the Physicians of Myddfai* (Pughe, 1861):

> §553 To prevent teeth becoming yellow and ill-smelling. Take the leaves of sage, powder with as much again of salt and make into balls. Bake them till they are burnt, and powder. Let your teeth be rubbed frequently therewith. It will render the teeth clean, white and sweet.

Commercially made herbal toothpastes containing sage are available in some health food shops, or use a daily mouthwash of sage each time you clean your teeth. Add 2 teaspoons of sage tincture to 250ml (½pt) of water and store in a clean bottle in the bathroom. Then use 5ml (1 teaspoonful) of this mixture with a little water as your daily mouth freshener. Modern studies suggest that rosmarinic acid (found in sage) can help to reduce dental plaque (van Dyke *et al.*, 1986).

WOUNDS

Sage is also one of our many wound herbs: apply a compress or poultice to slow-healing wounds.

CHAPTER 6

An Essential Approach

Essential oils from several species of sage are used in perfumery and for food flavourings, as well as in aromatherapy. Sage plants produce these aromatic oils in special secretory cells inside the leaves, and these substances then migrate to the surface of the leaf where they are stored adjacent to glandular hairs. Crushing a sage leaf between the fingers releases these potent substances and is a good way of becoming familiar with their distinctive smells.

Essential oils are most commonly collected by steam distillation. Steam is passed through a vat containing the plant material and dissolves the highly volatile oils (see diagram 3). This distillate is

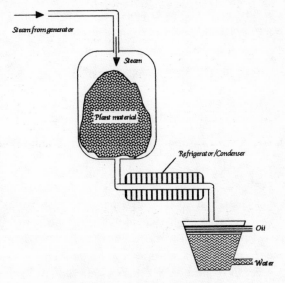

Diagram 3: Steam distillation.

then condensed in a cooler and collected. The oil, being lighter than water, floats to the surface and is easily skimmed off. In some cases the watery extract, known as a hydrolat in France, is also useful: rosewater and orange flower water are both made in this way although sage hydrolats are generally discarded.

Distillation has been used for extracting essential oils since at least the tenth century, while archaeological digs in Italy have also discovered crude stills, so the technique may have been known to the Romans.

Although technically quite simple, steam distillation is not a process for home use—yields are small and many tonnes of leaves and flowering tops are needed to produce viable commercial quantities of oil. Yields are typically 0.1–10 per cent—it takes 2,000kg (1¾ tons) of rose petals, for example, to produce just one kilo (2¼lb) of rose oil. An alternative for home use is to make an infused oil as described on p. 59.

Local variation

The same essential oils from plants grown in different areas often have slightly different chemical constituents depending on the type of soil, degree of sunshine, insect predators and so on. Yield and quality are also affected. In the past, these differences were considered to be minor and key therapeutic properties were believed to be much the same no matter where the material was collected.

Modern scientific analysis now suggests that the differences can, in fact, be so significant that properties and actions can vary markedly between members of the same species growing in different locations or even different altitudes.

The genetic make-up of the individual plant will also affect the oil. This is referred to as the 'chemotype' or 'botanical specificity' (bs) of the particular specimen. Increasingly, professional aromatherapists will specify a precise chemotype in addition to the species. Rosemary oil produced in Morocco, for example, is generally 'bs 1,8-cineole' (a chemical also found in high amounts in Greek sage oil); in the South of France rosemary oil is mostly 'bs camphor', while Spanish rosemary is generally 'bs bornyl acetate, verbenone'.

Sage oils are not usually further divided by chemotype although occasionally the dominant botanical specificity might be listed. This labelling system would be valuable if Greek sage and common sage were more widely differentiated instead of being generally sold in a blend. The botanical specificities given for commercially available sage oils are:

- *Salvia lavandulifolia* bs limonene (Spanish sage oil)
- *Salvia officinalis* bs thujones (common sage oil)
- *Salvia sclarea* bs linalyl acetate, sclareol (clary sage oil)

Using oils

Aromatic plant extracts, especially gums and resins, have been used in medicine since ancient times and a European perfumery industry, extracting oils much as we still do, certainly existed in the twelfth century. Oils are referred to in various mediaeval medical manuscripts, although modern aromatherapy was developed mainly in France in the 1920s by chemists like René-Maurice Gattefossé who published his classic text *Aromathérapie* in the 1930s (Gattefossé, 1937).

These early French aromatherapists placed great emphasis on the therapeutic actions of the 'aroma'—inhaling different scents which can have a direct impact on emotional well-being—and the French have also prescribed essential oils for internal use, taken in drop doses on lumps of sugar, or occasionally used in high concentrations in chest rubs and other highly focused external applications.

In the UK, essential oils are almost always used in external treatments: mostly in well diluted massage rubs by aromatherapists, added to baths or sometimes used in steam inhalations for nasal congestion. Until fairly recently British aromatherapy was considered by many as more of a relaxing type of beauty treatment than a reputable medical therapy. Essential oils are very potent medicine, however, and using them—even in dilute mixtures—purely as a beauty aid is both dangerous and misleading.

For home use it is best to use the essential oils externally only—

in massage, lotions, inhalations or baths; internal use needs skill and experience and is not recommended for home treatments.

While professional therapists may sometimes use concentrated oils, they really should be kept very dilute for home use. Typically, massage rubs are no more than 5 per cent oil [up to 5ml or 100 drops with 95ml (4fl oz) of carrier oil, such as almond or wheat germ] while only 5–10 drops of oil need be added to bathwater. A few drops of oil can also be added to simple skin creams or dispersed in a little vodka or distilled witch-hazel to make a lotion.

Constituents

Essential oils contain a complex cocktail of organic chemicals. There may be dozens in any one oil and in many cases they have not all been fully identified. These aromatic carbon-based compounds are classified by their structure and oxygen content—such as alcohols, ketones, aldehydes, phenols, acids and esters (table 3). In plants the basis molecular building block is a group of five linked carbon atoms (C_5); these build up to form large molecules known as terpenes—monoterpenes (C_{10}), sesquiterpenes (C_{15}) and diterpenes (C_{20}). Terpenes are compounds containing carbon (C) and hydrogen (H), while terpenoids also contain oxygen (O). The aromatic compounds found in essential oils are mainly terpenoids.

In general, aromatic aldehydes tend to be antiseptic, alcohols are tonic and stimulating, and ketones are usually toxic (Gattefossé, 1937). Since the 1930s, French aromatherapists have tried to classify these various groups of chemicals in terms of electrical energy—positive or negative—which phytotherapists like Pierre Franchomme (1985) equate with *yang* or *yin* activity. Negative or *yin* compounds are more passive, gentle and inwardly-focusing while the *yang* chemicals are more active, aggressive and outwardly moving. Franchomme sees aldehydes and esters as more *yin* in character, while alcohols and monoterpenes have a *yang* bias, with ketones in between (diagram 4, p. 78).

Clary sage, for example, is rich in acetates so is gentler and more *yin*, while common sage is richer in ketones and alcohols so is a more aggressive, *yang*-like oil.

Table 3: Categories of simple chemical constituents

GROUP	STRUCTURE	EXAMPLES
Alcohols	R–OH	linalol (lavender); borneol (sage and rosemary)
Aldehydes	$\begin{matrix} R \\ \searrow \\ H \nearrow \end{matrix} C{=}O$	citral (lemongrass)
Ketones	$\begin{matrix} R \\ \searrow \\ R^1 \nearrow \end{matrix} C{=}O$	carvone (caraway); thujone (sage)
Epoxides	$\begin{matrix} -C \\ | \\ -C \end{matrix} \!\!>\!\! O$	cineole (Spanish sage)
Phenols	(see structure)	eugenol (clove); thymol (thyme)
Esters	R–COOR^1	alkaloids such as atropine (deadly nightshade); linalyl acetate (clary sage)
Acids	R–COOH	citric acid (*Citrus* spp.); rosmarinic acid (sage and rosemary)

NB: R and R^1 represent alkyl groups such as CH_3—(methyl); C_2H_5—(ethyl) etc.

SPANISH SAGE OIL

Aroma: a pale yellow oil, rather fresher and more floral than common sage, with a hint of pine and lavender. Oils produced in the Middle East are often based on *S. fruticosa* rather than *S. lavandulifolia*, and have a high camphor content and distinct camphor-like aroma.

Principal constituents: camphor (up to 34 per cent), cineole (up to 35 per cent), limonene (up to 41 per cent), camphene (up to 20 per cent), pinene (up to 20 per cent).

77

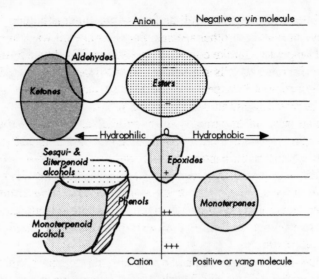

Diagram 4: Characters of essential oil molecules, according to
Pierre Franchomme.

Properties: antidepressant, anti-inflammatory, antimicrobial, antiseptic, antispasmodic, astringent, carminative, circulatory stimulant, deodorant, depurative, digestive, emmenagogue, expectorant,
febrifuge, hypotensive, nervine, oestrogenic effect, seborrhoeiac
regulator, stimulant for gall bladder and adrenal cortex, stomachic,
tonic, uterine stimulant.

Spanish sage oil is collected from steam distillation of the leaves.
Oil produced from leaves gathered early in the season tends to be
paler in colour, with darker, yellower oils being extracted from
late-harvested plants (Hilan *et al.*, 1997). Most production is, as
the name implies, in Spain from *S. lavandulifolia*, although *S.
fruticosa*, used in Turkey, Greece and other parts of the Middle
East, may also be marketed as Spanish sage oil.

Spanish sage oil is widely used in the perfumery industry for
scenting soaps and cosmetics and is also used for flavouring
drinks.

The Spanish regard sage oil as a cure-all and have traditionally
used it in washes to ward off infections or in lotions to soothe

insect bites and stings, as well as in rubs for rheumatic pains and digestive upsets. Like other species, Spanish sage oil was believed to give longevity. Unlike common sage (see p. 80), concentrations of toxic thujones in oils marked as 'Spanish sage' are very low, typically between 0.72 per cent and 1.86 per cent, compared with the 50 per cent found in common sage plants.

Spanish sage oil is strongly antimicrobial; recent studies with Greek sage oil (Hilan *et al.*, 1997) have demonstrated its particular efficacy against such bacteria as *Klebsiella ozaenae*, *Morganella morganii*, *Staphylococcus* spp., *Streptococcus* spp, and *Candida albicans*. Even at low concentrations this oil was more efficient at killing these bacteria than commercial antibiotics, although it was less effective against *Pseudomonas aeriginosa*, *E. coli* and *Salmonella typhi*.

Studies also show that Spanish sage oil can combat antibiotic-resistant germs (Yehia and Marth, 1993), suggesting that it could become even more important as these bacteria proliferate.

This antimicrobial activity makes Spanish sage oil especially useful in external treatment for boils, skin infections, cuts and grazes, as a general antiseptic, or in gargles and mouthwashes for laryngitis and gum infections. Traditionally, aromatherapists also use the oil in massage treatments for aches and pains, circulation problems, digestive weaknesses, colds and 'flu.

CAUTION: Although Spanish sage oil is relatively non-toxic and non-irritant, it should still be completely avoided in pregnancy and used in moderation at other times.

USING SPANISH SAGE OIL

Acne: Add 10 drops of oil to 50ml (2fl oz) of rosewater and 50ml (2fl oz) of distilled witch hazel and use to bathe acne pustules.

Aches and pains: Add 5 drops of oil to a teaspoon of almond oil and massage into aching muscles and joints or for arthritis and rheumatism.

Chest rubs: Add 5 drops of oil to a teaspoon of almond oil and use to massage the chest and throat in cases of asthma, bronchitis and laryngitis.

Colds, 'flu and catarrh: Use the chest rub (above), or add 3–4 drops of oil to a basin of boiling water and use as a steam inhalation.

Cuts and grazes: Add 5 drops of oil to half a cup of hot water to clean cuts and grazes; apply a dressing if required. The same mix can be used to bathe skin sores.

Dandruff: Add 20 drops of oil to 500ml (1pt) of warm water and use as a final rinse after shampooing the hair. Spanish sage is also said to combat hair loss: add 2 drops to a teaspoon of almond oil and massage into the scalp each night.

Excessive sweating: Add 10 drops of oil to 250ml (½pt) of water in a plastic spray bottle and use as an antiperspirant.

Gargles: Add 2 drops of oil to a cup of warm water and use as a gargle for sore throat, laryngitis, tonsillitis or pharyngitis; do not swallow the wash after rinsing your mouth but spit it out.

Gum infections and gingivitis: Add 2 drops of oil to half a cup of warm water and use as a mouthwash night and morning; do not swallow the wash after rinsing your mouth but spit it out.

Headaches: Add 2 drops of oil to a teaspoon of almond oil and use to massage the nape of the neck, temples or between the eyes to ease head pains.

Period pains/menstrual cramps: Add 2 drops of oil to a teaspoon of almond oil and use as an abdominal massage to ease cramping pains. Repeat every 3–4 hours if need be.

Poor circulation: Add 5 drops of oil to bathwater to help stimulate poor circulation; alternatively add 5 drops to water in a footbath or handbath to stimulate peripheral circulation and soak for 10–15 minutes or until the water cools.

Stress: Spanish sage oil can be helpful for nervous exhaustion and stress-related disorders—add 5 drops to a warm bath or use 2 drops in a teaspoon of almond oil and ask a friend to massage your shoulders and back.

COMMON SAGE OIL

Aroma: a pale yellow oil with a warm, spicy, camphor-like smell. Popular in perfumery.

Principal constituents: α- and β-thujone (up to 50 per cent), cineole, borneol, salviol, caryophyllene and other terpenes.

Properties: anti-inflammatory, antibacterial, antifungal, antioxidant, antiseptic, antispasmodic, astringent, digestive, diuretic, emmenagogue, febrifuge, hypertensive, insecticide, laxative, stomachic, tonic.

Common sage oil is collected by steam distillation of the leaves and flowering tops: experts are said to prefer 'small-leaved' specimens which produce a greater oil yield than larger-leaved plants—which may suggest that *S. fruticosa* is being used rather than *S. officinalis*. The oil is more popular in perfumery than Spanish sage oil as it has a more refined and focused scent.

Sage oil is extremely toxic due to the high proportion of thujones which can trigger fits in epileptics, cause convulsions and have a range of very unpleasant side-effects. The French phytotherapist Jean Valnet (1964) describes the oil as 'two times more toxic than absinthe'—a potent alcoholic drink flavoured with wormwood (*Artemisia absinthium*) extract which has been known to lead to blindness and insanity and has been banned in many countries, starting with Switzerland in 1908.

Many professional aromatherapists, such as Patricia Davis (1988), have reported numerous cases, at first hand, of patients who have suffered from sage poisoning, generally after attempting self-treatment. Symptoms can include violent abdominal pain, severe uterine contractions and very heavy menstrual bleeding. In each case the sage oil had been used in massage or baths at a dose of 2–10 drops.

This high level of toxicity means that many British aromatherapists avoid sage oil and prefer to use clary sage instead. In France, however, the oil is prescribed for internal use, taken in doses of 2 to 4 drops, three times a day, mixed with a teaspoonful of honey.

Great caution is needed in any home use of sage oil as everyone is different and adverse reactions have been reported in doses as low as two drops. It is best avoided by the untrained—especially as other, safer oils can be just as effective. It is sometimes used, very well diluted, to massage the abdomen during the early stages of labour to help stimulate contractions. Recent studies (Jalsenjak *et al.*, 1987; Janssen, 1989) have confirmed its strong antimicrobial properties, so even if it is regarded as too toxic for use in home first aid it would certainly be effective as a household disinfectant! [Use 20 drops to 500ml (1pt) of water to wash kitchen and bathroom surfaces, or in spray bottles as a lavatory cleaner.]

Philippe Mailhebiau (1995) describes sage oil as a 'huntress'— a strong, energetic remedy for seeking out and clearing obstructions. 'Its might,' he says, 'must be appreciated for it to be used wisely since it can go from being a saving to a destructive essence changing from a regulator of the hormonal function into a haemorrhagic, abortifacient product.' He recommends blending sage oil with *Ravensara aromatica* and *Melaleuca quinquenervia* for treating genital herpes, or combining it with rosemary oil for bedsores—both serious conditions for which amateur home treatment should not be attempted.

Although sage oil is generally described as warming, it can be an effective remedy (like common sage itself) for excessive sweating and can also be helpful if the problem is foul-smelling sweat; 2–3 drops of oil in a 250ml (½pt) plastic spray bottle of water can make an effective antiperspirant. Similar dilutions could be used as a mouth spray for gum disorders or mouth ulcers, or it can be added to mouthwashes and gargles as an alternative to the tincture or tea (see chapter 5). Use no more than two drops in half a tumbler of warm water and, unlike gargles made from tea or tincture, do not swallow the mixture.

It is worth learning the smells of Spanish sage and common sage oil as there is often confusion with labelling in poor-quality commercial supplies. However, the common confusion of both plants with *S. fruticosa* does little to help the purity of supplies.

CAUTION: Never underestimate the potential toxicity of sage oil; use only as suggested for sprays and mouthwashes and stop immediately if any side-effects occur. Avoid completely in pregnancy or if trying to conceive.

CLARY SAGE OIL

Aroma: sweet, strong, floral, slightly nutty scent—Philippe Mailhebiau (1995) describes it as 'a feeling of something unfinished, like fruit that is still green'.

Principal constituents: linalyl acetate (up to 75 per cent), linalol, pinene, myrcene, phellandrine; constituents vary significantly according to geographic origin.

Properties: antibacterial, anticonvulsive, antidepressant, antiseptic, antispasmodic, aphrodisiac, astringent, carminative, deodorant, digestive, emmenagogue, hypotensive, nervine, seborrhoeic regulator, sedative, tonic, uterine stimulant.

Clary sage oil is collected by steam distillation of the flowering tops and leaves. The yield can be as low as 0.05 per cent which makes it difficult to produce, so good-quality oil can be expensive: French growers call it 'night beauty' as its fragrant evening scent seems to slip away by morning. It is a popular essence in the perfumery market, used in scents and soaps, while its muscatel flavour makes it valuable as a food essence and it is often used in the drinks industry to flavour wines.

As well as the essential oil, clary sage is available as a 'concrete'—a concentrated waxy, solid perfume material extracted from the plant using hexane (a hydrocarbon solvent); and as an 'absolute' which is a highly concentrated viscous semi-solid, extracted from the concrete using alcohol.

Unlike common sage and Spanish sage oils, clary does not contain any toxic compounds (α- and β-thujone or borneone) however, inevitable uninformed confusion means that clary is often grouped with these other sages and held to be toxic.

The plant is rich in esters rather than the ketones of common sage, so that it is primarily rebalancing and antispasmodic. It is ideal for combating both depression and overexcitability and it works at a deep level, acting as a restorative for emotional and spiritual problems.

Like its relatives, clary sage oil is also excellent for gynaecological problems such as amenorrhoea, dysmenorrhoea and vaginal discharges (leucorrhoea). Some French aromatherapists recommend combining it with low doses of common sage oil to enhance the effect, but given the toxicity this is not something for amateur experiment. Clary sage oil can both slow down and encourage menstrual flow depending on the predisposition of the patient—which, Philippe Mailhebiau argues, confirms the 'intelligence of essential oils'. He maintains that it is also useful at puberty 'to help women cross the barrier from barrenness to fertility'. In the same way it can be an appropriate choice at the menopause to combat depression, although it becomes less relevant in old age. Combining clary sage oil massage rubs with common sage tea is a nice way to capitalise on the benefits of both herbs during the menopause.

Mailhebiau claims that clary sage also works well with oregano oil (*Origanum majorana*) for psychological problems in young girls; with dill and basil oils as an antispasmodic for back pains associated with menstruation; or with petitgrain oil (distilled from the leaves of bitter orange—*Citrus aurantium*) for sleep disturbances associated with heartache. He sees clary as a 'young girl stepping into womanhood, an adolescent torn between childhood and adulthood and inner femininity which she has yet to learn how to assert in everyday life'. While he equates common sage oil with Artemis, the huntress of Greek mythology, he personifies clary as Eos, the young goddess of the dawn.

Others describe clary sage oil as 'euphoric'—although not everyone becomes quite so excited by its smell, and some people simply find the oil very calming and relaxing, leading to drowsiness and sleep. Robert Tisserand (1977) describes the effect as 'more like cannabis than alcohol'.

Clary sage oil is generally regarded as mildly hypotensive to reduce blood pressure (Rovesti and Gattefossé, 1973). It will also stimulate the adrenal cortex, so may be helpful for those recovering from a course of steroidal therapy.

CAUTION: Avoid clary sage oil in pregnancy and when drinking alcohol as it can enhance the effect. Avoid driving after using clary sage in massage treatments.

USING CLARY SAGE OIL

Acne: Add 20 drops of oil to 50ml (2fl oz) of rosewater and 50ml of distilled witch-hazel and use to bathe acne pustules.

Asthma: Clary sage can be especially helpful in asthma. Make a chest rub by adding 10 drops of oil to a teaspoon of almond oil and use to massage the chest area during mild attacks and as a preventative. The same remedy can also be used for whooping cough. In both these ailments professional treatment is recommended and clary should be used to support other medication, not replace it.

Boils: Put 3 drops of oil and 6 drops of water onto a cotton swab or lint and fasten over the boil with sticking plaster to encourage it to discharge. Repeat every 2–3 hours as need be.

Dandruff, oily hair and hair loss: Add 20 drops of oil to 500ml (1pt) of warm water and use as a final rinse after shampooing the hair. Clary sage is said to be especially effective as a rinse for greasy or oily hair. Like Spanish sage, it also reputedly combats hair loss: add 2 drops to a teaspoon of almond oil and massage into the scalp each night.

Depression: Clary sage oil is used by professional aromatherapists to treat debility and depression. Because of its soporific effect it is best used in relaxing, tonic baths each evening: Add 3–5 drops to the bathwater.

Digestive upsets: Clary is warming and antispasmodic so can help to relieve griping, colicky pains. Add 2–3 drops to a teaspoon of almond oil and massage the abdominal area. The same treatment can also be helpful for indigestion and flatulence.

Frigidity/loss of libido: Clary sage is a reputed aphrodisiac, largely because of its slightly intoxicating and euphoric property. It can be used in mutual massage between partners before making love—dilute 5 drops in 2 teaspoons of almond oil and take turns to massage back, chest and abdomen.

Menstrual problems: Use as Spanish sage (p. 80) for menstrual cramps and period pains. Clary can also be helpful for amenorrhoea—use 2 drops of oil in a teaspoon of almond oil as a daily abdominal massage between periods. For vaginal discharges (leucorrhoea) use 10 drops to 250ml (½pt) of water in a douche, or the same mixture in a plastic spray bottle and use to spray the vagina and perineum.

Tonic: Clary is a good general tonic for the nervous system, kidneys, stomach and uterus. It can be used in regular massage or baths—add 5 drops to a warm bath or use 2 drops in a teaspoon of almond oil and ask a friend to massage your shoulders and back. As a mild hypotensive it can also be helpful for stress-related high blood pressure.

CHAPTER 7

Sage Goes East

There is a tradition that in the seventeenth century Dutch traders would happily exchange two or three cases of European sage for a chest of Chinese tea (*Camellia sinensis*) and thought they were getting the better deal. The Chinese simply regarded this as yet another example of Western stupidity, since they knew that sage was a far more valuable herb.

As well as having a high regard for European sage, the Chinese use their own oriental member of the *Salvia* family, *Dan Shen* (*Salvia miltiorrhiza*), which today is cultivated commercially in Central China. The name *Dan Shen* literally means 'scarlet root' and the herb is sold either as solid roots with its distinctive red bark or in thin, washed slices. The Chinese have used *Dan Shen* as an invigorating blood tonic for at least 3,000 years. First mention of the plant is in the *Shen Nong Ban Cao Jing* or 'the divine farmer's classic herbal':

> *Dan Shen* is bitter and slightly cold. It is non-toxic, treating mainly evil *Qi* in the heart and abdomen, continual gurgling of the intestines like water running, cold and heat, and gatherings and accumulations. It breaks concretions and eliminates conglomerations, relieves vexatious fullness and boosts the *Qi*. Its other name is *Que Chan Cao* (Cicada-deterring weed). It grows in mountains and valleys. (Yang, 1998)

This book takes its name from the legendary figure of Shen Nong, one of the three founding emperors of China, who first taught mankind how to cultivate grains and is reputed to have personally tasted hundreds of herbs to identify their healing properties. Shen

87

Nong had succeeded Fu Xi, who gave the Chinese a universal philosophy to interpret and explain all natural phenomena, and he was followed in his turn by Huang Di, the Yellow Emperor, the supreme ruler of the universe, who introduced music, medicine and mathematics, writing and weapons.

Shen Nong reputedly lived some time between 4000 and 2500 BC, although the *Shen Nong Ban Cao Jing*—believed to encapsulate much older traditions—is generally dated to around 500 BC.

In Chinese medicine *Dan Shen* is usually described as 'invigorating the Blood and breaking up congealed Blood', which to Western ears makes it sound like some sort of anticoagulant or circulatory stimulant. It does both—but that is only part of the story as the Chinese mean rather more by 'Blood' than simply the red stuff found in our veins and arteries.

TRADITIONAL CHINESE MEDICINE

Traditional Chinese medicine is based on the ancient Taoist principles, dating back to Fu Xi, of the 'five elements' and the importance of harmony between *yin* and *yang*. Just as the ancient Greeks

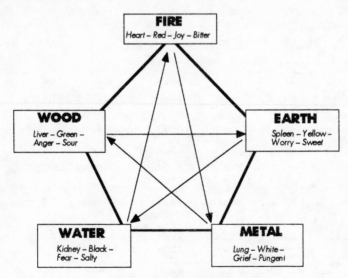

Diagram 5: The Five Element Model.

believed that all things were composed of earth, air, water and fire, so the Chinese applied similar logic and decided that all matter was made up of earth, metal, water, wood and fire.

These elements were not only closely interrelated, influencing and controlling each other (see diagram 5), but they were also matched to a lengthy series of other phenomena, all grouped in fives—five solid body organs, five emotions, five seasons and so on (see table 4). It was important to maintain balance between these five elements as any overexuberance or weakness would affect the inner harmony: if Water, related to the Kidney, is weak, for example, then it can fail to control Fire which will then attack Metal, associated with the Lung, so leading to respiratory problems.

As well as this five element model, early Chinese physicians also saw well-being and illness in terms of *yin* and *yang*—two basic creative forces central to all things. *Yin* and *yang* have been

Table 4: Five Phase associations

	WOOD	FIRE	EARTH	METAL	WATER
Direction:	East	South	Centre	West	North
Colour:	Green	Red	Yellow	White	Black
Season:	Spring	Summer	Late Summer (traditionally from c. July 7 for a month)	Autumn	Winter
Climate:	Wind	Hot	Dampness	Dryness	Cold
Solid organ (*Zang*):	Liver	Heart	Spleen	Lung	Kidney
Hollow organ (*Fu*):	Gall Bladder	Small Intestine	Stomach	Large Intestine	Urinary Bladder
Sense organs/ openings:	Eyes Sight	Tongue Speech	Mouth Taste	Nose Smell	Ears Hearing
Emotion:	Anger	Joy/Fright	Worry	Sadness/Grief	Fear
Taste:	Sour	Bitter	Sweet	Pungent/Acrid	Salty
Tissues:	Tendon Nails	Blood vessels Complexion	Muscles Lips	Skin Body hair	Bone Head hair
Sound:	Shouting	Laughing	Singing	Weeping	Groaning
Smell:	Rancid	Burnt	Fragrant	Rotten	Putrid
Body fluid:	Tears	Sweat	Saliva	Mucus	Urine
Meat:	Chicken	Mutton	Beef	Horse	Pork
Cereal:	Wheat	Glutinous millet	Millet	Rice	Beans

NB: In order to differentiate the complex Chinese organ concepts from our Western anatomy, it is customary to give them initial capitals.

89

compared to the light and dark sides of the mountain, the above and below, or the outside and inside; essentially they are paired and inseparable opposites, vital to all things and contained within all things.

Both aspects are always present at all times although the balance shifts from time to time. Summer, for example, is more strongly *yang* as it is a hot, bright season but it still contains some *yin*, while damp and cold winter is more closely aligned with *yin*, although it still contains a remnant of *yang*. The same concepts are applied in traditional Chinese medicine to the human body, so that substances (static things) are seen as more *yin* while functions (activities) are more *yang*: organs, blood and body fluids thus tend to be *yin* while the functions—transporting and transforming things as with breathing and digestion—are seen as more *yang*.

Fundamental substances

As well as the groups of solid and hollow organs, each with their complex set of physical, emotional and spiritual attributes, the 'fundamental substances' are central to traditional Chinese medicine. These control many bodily functions and are essential for life. The five substances are:

- *Jing* or 'essence', which is the source of living organisms and the most important of this group of life materials. *Jing* is stored in the Kidney and is associated with both reproduction and creativity. We are each born with a store of essential 'congenital *Jing*' which gradually decays during our lives. This steady erosion is the main cause, in Chinese theory, for such symptoms of ageing as hearing loss, greying hair and the menopause.
- *Qi* or 'vital energy', which has become a familiar concept in the West. Its main characteristic is motion, the activity of life. There are numerous varieties of *Qi*, including defence energy (*Wei Qi*) which can be equated with the immune system, primordial *Qi* (*Yuan Qi*) which is with us from birth, and nourishing *Qi* (*Ying Qi*), largely

90

produced from the energy of our food. *Ying Qi* is collected and transformed in the Spleen, becoming part of the Blood, and supplying nutrients throughout the body.

- *Jin-Ye* or 'body fluids', which includes substances such as saliva, gastric juices, phlegm, tears, mucus and sweat.
- *Shen* which is usually translated as 'spirit', the inner vitality closely associated with human consciousness. It is associated with the Heart and is also sometimes described as 'awareness'—a full consciousness of surroundings, actions and capabilities.
- *Xue* or 'Blood', which is believed to be formed from a mixture of nourishing *Qi* (*Ying Qi*), food essence and body fluids.

While the concept of *Xue* encompasses the familiar red fluid that courses through our veins, it also goes a little further. Blood is regarded as essential for mental activities, so that if *Xue* and *Qi* are strong, the person will be clear-thinking and vigorous; if these substances are weak then the individual may have problems in concentrating. Similarly, the link with body fluids means that activities like sweating, which may damage *Jin-Ye*, are also regarded as damaging to the Blood. The Chinese also believe that the Liver stores Blood, so any damage to the Liver is likely to harm Blood, while weak Liver *Qi* will lead to Blood stagnation.

Because Blood and body fluids are regarded as predominantly *yin* in nature, any illness involving dryness, a lack of sweating or a blood weakness might be seen as involving *yin* deficiency.

BLOOD DISORDERS
In traditional Chinese pathology there are four major syndromes which can affect *Xue* (Blood):

- bleeding or haemorrhage
- stagnant or congealed blood
- heat attacking the blood
- deficient blood

Dan Shen is traditionally included with the group of herbs used to combat congealed or stagnant blood—usually described as 'invigorating' the blood.

'Stagnant Blood' syndrome occurs when the flow of blood is blocked or the blood becomes static. This may be the result of external pathogens, be caused by inappropriate treatment of haemorrhage, by traumatic injury, by stagnation of *Qi*, or—in women—by retention of the lochia following childbirth (Yanchi, 1988). Stagnant blood is characterised by a fixed pain which is not eased by either hot compresses or ice packs, and typical signs include purplish skin, dark purple lips and dry scaly skin.

Distinct conditions in modern medicine like thrombosis, local ischaemia, menstrual problems, certain heart disorders or haemorrhage might all be classified in traditional Chinese medicine (TCM) as aspects of congealed blood.

Dan Shen is one of the most important herbs for treating stagnant blood. Others that are widely used include *Chuan Xiong* (Szechuan lovage root—*Ligusticum wallachii*) and *Yu Jin* (turmeric—*Curcuma longa*).

USING *DAN SHEN*

In Chinese medicine, herbs are traditionally described in terms of their characteristic taste, temperature (hot, cold or neutral) and the parts of the body which they affect. Tastes include sour, astringent, bitter, sweet, pungent/acrid, salty or bland and these can also be related back to the five element model as an indication of other likely characteristics of the plant. *Dan Shen* is described in modern Chinese herbals as bitter and slightly cold, and it particularly affects the Heart, Liver and Pericardium (the sac around the heart).

In China the roots are collected between November and March—although early November is considered the best time. They are trimmed, washed and sun dried. Once clean the root crown is removed, and the roots wrapped in a moist cloth and left until they are uniformly damp; they are then cut into thin slices and once more dried in the sun.

The character and properties of Chinese herbs can be subtly altered by cooking or soaking the plant material in various ways:

- *Dan Shen* is used in its crude form for invigorating the blood and clearing stagnation.
- Roasted *Dan Shen* is made by stir-frying the roots over a low flame until around 5 per cent of the surface is charcoaled: it is used as a styptic to stop bleeding, and stir-fried with rice it is used as a harmonising remedy for the stomach. Stir-frying with wine enhances the general effect of the herb.
- Rather less savoury is cooking the root with turtle's blood to make a remedy focused on the liver, or stir-fried with pig's blood to shift the emphasis to the heart and increase the calming effect on the spirit.

In China *Dan Shen* is the herb of choice for treating heart problems such as angina pectoris and coronary heart disease which may be associated with stagnant Blood. In Chinese theory the Liver is involved with regulating the menstrual cycle, so it is no surprise that *Dan Shen* (which affects the Liver meridian) is a key herb for stagnant blood problems in the lower abdomen—the sort of disorders which in the West we would term dysmenorrhoea (period pain) or amenorrhoea (absence of periods). Because it is also cooling, *Dan Shen* is used for problems associated with heat and toxins in the blood, which the Chinese would see as the cause of boils and skin ulcers. Similarly, because the Heart is also associated with the spirit and mental activity (see table 4), the combined cooling aspect and heart focus of *Dan Shen* make it suitable as a sedative or tranquilliser, given for insomnia, irritability and palpitations.

While these attributes date back long before the days of chemical analysis and modern pathology, modern trials do suggest that *Dan Shen* is effective in all these ways. As well as its action on the circulatory system, it has been shown to lower blood sugar and blood cholesterol levels, increase metabolism and stimulate the immune system.

Known ingredients include a series of diterpene diketones (tan-

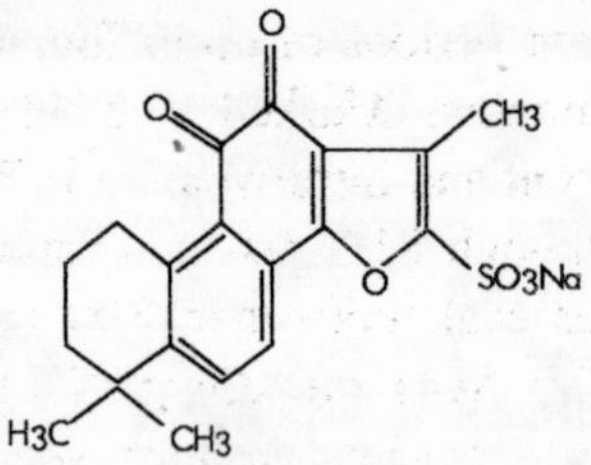

Diagram 6: Water soluble tanshinone II sodium sulphate.

shinones, cryptotanshinone, isotanshinone, miltirone, and isocryptotanshinone) as well as the salviol found in common sage (Yeung, 1985; Yen, 1992). The main component is tanshinone 2A (up to 0.05 per cent, see diagram 6). Unlike common sage, however, it has no oestrogenic effect, nor does it contain toxic thujones.

Dan Shen and the heart

Decoctions of the herb have been shown in animal studies to improve coronary blood flow and combat the effects of myocardial infarction, dilate the coronary blood vessels and peripheral blood vessels, so helping to reduce blood pressure, increase blood flow— especially in the microcirculation (Chang and But, 1986)—and also to enhance the activity of other cardiotonic herbs to improve cardiac output (Zhu *et al.*, 1987).

As one might expect of a plant traditionally used to clear stagnant blood, it also has an anticoagulant effect, largely due to tanshinone-related compounds, and will reduce the size of blood clots and clotting time (Wang *et al.*, 1989). Animal studies suggest that *Dan Shen* can prevent intramicrovascular coagulation, so relieving local anaemia and lack of blood flow affecting the surrounding tissues. The herb can also enhance the effect of conventional anticoagulant treatments such as warfarin (Lo *et al.*, 1992).

There have been a number of studies in this area in recent years which have demonstrated that *Dan Shen* can be very effective for combating a range of heart and circulatory disorders. One widely reported trial involved 323 patients suffering from angina pectoris, who were given the equivalent of 60g (2½oz) of *Dan Shen* three times daily in treatment periods of up to four weeks, repeated for from one to nine months. Marked clinical improvement was recorded in 14.8 per cent and improvement in 38.4 per cent, based on ECG findings, although 81.3 per cent reported a reduction in symptoms. In another trial more than 300 patients with angina pectoris were given *Dan Shen* with *Jiang Xiang* (*Dalbergia odorifera*), with 50 per cent recording an improvement in ECG results and 82 per cent claiming a reduction in symptoms (Bensky and Gamble, 1986; Foster and Chongxi, 1992).

Other studies have shown that *Dan Shen* injections can reduce mortality from heart attacks from 39 per cent to 13 per cent if treatment is given within 24 hours, and it has also been used in a similar way in combination with other herbs with good results (Keji, 1981; Guo *et al.*, 1983).

Specific reports on *Dan Shen* usage from Chinese hospitals include an analysis of 110 elderly patients suffering from cerebral thrombosis, who were given *Dan Shen* in combination with *Huang Qi* (*Astragalus membranaceus*), *Chuan Xiong* (Szechuan lovage root, *Ligusticum wallachii*) and *Chi Shao* (red peony, *Paeonia lactiflora*) for 28 days: 47.3 per cent were claimed to have made a 'complete cure' while 32.7 per cent showed a 'marked improvement'. The researchers (Zhang *et al.*, 1982) argued that the cause of the disease was deficiency of Blood and *Qi*, and poor circulation leading to Blood and *Qi* stagnation.

The herb has also been used in trials involving patients suffering from cerebral atherosclerosis—a common cause of dizziness and confusion in the elderly. In a small-scale test, 26 from a total of 42 patients were deemed 'cured', while a further 11 showed significant improvement using a range of remedies selected to match the likely cause of their problems. The researchers concluded that *Dan Shen* was most effective where causes included:

- deficiency of *Qi* and Blood complicated by Blood stagnation
- deficiency of *yin* and *Jing*
- stagnation of phlegm and Blood (Li *et al.*, 1987)

Dan Shen and menstrual problems

Dan Shen is traditionally used for period pain, absence of menstruation or for lower abdominal pain associated with endometriosis and other gynaecological disorders. As a rule it is used in wine for menstrual problems, which in Chinese theory helps to make the plant rather more warming.

Studies involving the use of the herb in gynaecological conditions include one project (Lin, 1983) in which *Dan Shen* was the primary herb used in a trial of 126 women suffering from a range of disorders, among them uterine bleeding, sterility and period paid. In Western medicine these ailments would never be considered as a homogeneous group for a clinical trial, but in traditional medicine all can be treated using the therapeutic principle of *Huo Xue Huayu*—promoting Blood circulation and removing blood stasis.

In this study severe uterine bleeding associated with complications from childbirth or endometriosis was stopped in an average of 3.8 days by using a combination of *Dan Shen* with tree peony (*Paeonia suffruticosa*), red peony (*P. lactiflora*), peach seeds (*Prunus persica*), safflower (*Carthamus tinctorius*), Chinese motherwort (*Leonurus sibiricus*), notoginseng (*Panax pseudoginseng*) and nutgrass (*Cyperus rotundus*).

Other properties

As well as its established uses in heart and menstrual problems, research has also shown that *Dan Shen* is cardioprotective, hypotensive, anticoagulant, antiplatelet, fibrinolytic, hepato-protective, vulnerary, antifibrotic and antibacterial. Tests have shown that it will combat a variety of bacteria including *Staphylococcus aureus*, *E. coli*, *Shigella dysenteriae* and *Mycobacterium tuberculosis* (Bensky and Gamble, 1986; Yeung, 1985). Extracts also show some cytoxic (anticancer) activity in laboratory experiments (Bone, 1996).

The key antibacterial component is believed to be cryptotanshinone which has been isolated and given in tablets or ointments for tonsillitis, infected sores and other bacterial problems. The major constituents are water soluble and infusions have been effectively used as an antifungal wash.

Dan Shen is also sedating and will prolong the effect of barbiturates. It shows antioxidant activity and there are suggestions that it can help repair liver lesions while enriching liver-cell nutrition (Foster and Chongxi, 1992). In studies it has proved effective in the treatment of chronic hepatitis, used in conjunction with *Hypericum japonicum* (Chang and But, 1986), or with turmeric and Chinese hawthorn (*Crataegus pinnatifida*) (Liao *et al.*, 1987). A study involving 176 patients suffering from acute hepatitis—using a mixture of *Dan Shen* with woad (*Isatis tinctoria*), evergreen wormwood (*Artemisia scoparia*), red peony (*Paeonia lactiflora*) tree peony (*Paeonia suffruticosa*) and several other Chinese herbs—reported a complete cure rate of 89.8 per cent (Wang, 1987).

DAN SHEN PREPARATIONS

Typical accepted dosage for *Dan Shen* is 2–6g of dried root daily. However, most reports of its use in Chinese journals recommend at least 10–30g (up to 1oz) of the herb daily.

In Chinese medicine, herbs are very rarely used singly; instead they are combined in traditional formulae which have evolved over the centuries. Chinese medical students must learn hundreds of these prescriptions by heart, much as Western students learn to recite the names of muscles and bones. Each formula is deemed appropriate for a particular disease syndrome and *Dan Shen* features in several which are used for Blood stagnation and Heat syndromes.

Among the more important formulae including *Dan Shen* are:

Dan Shen Yin which contains:
Dan Shen 15–30g
Tan Xiang (sandalwood, *Santalum album*) 3–6g
Sha Ren (bastard cardomum, *Amomum xanthioides*) 3–6g
This is made into a decoction or soup with water and is a

classic formula to invigorate Blood and *Qi* circulation and relieve pain and Blood stasis. It is mainly prescribed for angina pectoris.

Jia Wei Mai Men Dong Tang which contains:
   Mai Men Dong (Japanese hyacinth, *Ophiopogon japonicus*) 9–15g
   Shan Yao (Chinese yam, *Dioscorea opposita*) 9–12g
   Ren Shen (Korean ginseng, *Panax ginseng*) 9–12g
   Dan Shen 9–12g
   Ban Xia (*Pinellia ternata*) 6–9g
   Bai Shao (white peony, *Paeonia lactiflora*) 6–9g
   Tao Ren (peach stones, *Prunus persica*) 3–6g
   Da Zao (Chinese dates, *Ziziphus jujube*) 3–5 pieces
   Gan Cao (Chinese liquorice, *Glycyrrhiza uralensis*) 3–6g
This is made up into decoction and is used for menstrual irregularities, especially if there are also digestive upsets or nosebleeds associated with the menstrual cycle.

Qing Ying Tang which contains:
   Sheng Di Huang (raw Chinese foxglove, *Rehmannia glutinosa*) 10–15g
   Xuan Shen (Chinese figwort, *Scrophularia ningpoensis*) 6–9g
   Mai Men Dong (Japanese hyacinth, *Ophiopogon japonicus*) 6–9g
   Zhu Ye (bamboo leaf, *Phyllostachys nigra*) 3–6g
   Huang Lian (Chinese golden thread, *Coptis chinensis*) 1–3g
   Jin Yin Hua (honeysuckle flowers, *Lonicera japonica*) 6–9g
   Lian Qiao (forsythia berries, *Forsythia suspensa*) 6–9g
   Dan Shen 3–6g
Traditionally it also includes rhinoceros horn, although few Westerners would endorse this cruel use of an endangered animal. *Qing Ying Tang* is a cooling combination which is used for a variety of toxic heat syndromes, such as septicaemia and epidemic meningitis, and also to nourish *yin*.

Formulations like these—with their occasional rather unsavoury ingredients—have been virtually unchanged for hundreds of years.

They generally originate from the work of early physicians, such as *Prescriptions of the Golden Chamber* (*Jingui Yaolue*) written by Zhang Zhongjing (*c.* AD 150–219), and the exact proportions will be slightly adjusted by an experienced practitioner to reflect the needs of individual patients.

Herbs often used in simpler combinations with *Dan Shen* by modern practitioners include:

- *Dang Gui* (*Angelica polymorpha* var. *sinensis*) for menstrual irregularities;
- *Mu Dan Pi* (tree peony, *Paeonia suffruticosa*) and *Sheng Di Huang* (*Rehmannia glutinosa*) for fevers and irritability;
- *Suan Zao Ren* (*Zizyphus jujuba*) and *Bai Zi Ren* (*Thuja orientalis*) for palpitations and insomnia.

Combinations based on some of these classic prescriptions are now available in the West, prepared as neatly packaged pills or tinctures to meet European tastes. Well-known TCM expert Ted Kaptchuk, for example, uses *Dan Shen* in his 'Compassionate Sage' remedy to calm disturbed *Shen* (Fratkin, 1986) while Giovanni Maciocia (1995) has included *Dan Shen* in several of his 'Three Treasures' remedies, among them 'Red Stirring' (prescribed to move Blood stasis in the Heart) and 'Stir Field of Elixir' (to clear Blood stasis in the lower abdomen). The Shanghai Chinese Medicines Works sells *Dan Shen* in tablet form (75 per cent) with borneol crystals (a stimulating terpenoid alcohol found in rosemary, common sage and other herbs).

Making remedies

Chinese herbal remedies are traditionally made up into soups or *Tang*—brewed in a large crockery pot kept in each household especially for the purpose.

The herbal mixture is dispensed by the Chinese herbal pharmacy in a series of paper bags—one for each daily dose. This is then boiled in three cups of water in the *Tang* pot for 25–30 minutes until the liquid has reduced by half. The mix is then strained and taken in a single dose on an empty stomach in the morning. The same herbs might be used for the following day's brew depending on the exact mix: if it contains soluble ingredients such as certain mineral salts, then a fresh prescription will be needed each day.

The *Tang* is generally very dark brown and very strongly flavoured: few Westerners find the brews even remotely palatable, and although many chronic sufferers are willing to make and take their medicines in the traditional way, others find the whole process incompatible with Western lifestyles—which, of course, may be a factor in their particular health problems.

Using *Dan Shen* at home

Chinese herbs are often subject to adulteration and mislabelling, so always buy from a reputable supplier—even Chinatown herbalists get it wrong sometimes—or ask a qualified TCM practitioner to check the material for you. Alternatively use tinctures or powdered *Dan Shen* from a reputable (preferably Western, Japanese or Singapore) source.

Crude *Dan Shen* is reddish brown and usually sold in the West in pieces around 5–8cm (2–3in) long. It is available both as the dried herb or made up into a tincture (an alcohol/water extract) and sold in dropper bottles. Prepared tinctures like this can be highly priced and often the drop doses recommended are far below anything the Chinese would consider of therapeutic value. To produce your own, follow the instructions for making tinctures given on p. 56, although it is worth remembering that *Dan Shen* in wine or alcohol is better for menstrual problems than for cardiovascular disorders.

To use the herb as a simple, brew 15g (½oz) in two cups of water for 20 minutes, strain the liquid and take in a single daily dose.

A nice way to take Chinese roots is in tonic wines: fill a vinegar vat with the dried herb, cover completely with red wine and leave for two weeks. Then draw off sherry glass doses of the brew from the tap at the bottom of the vat each day. Continue to add more red wine to keep the herb completely covered, otherwise it will go mouldy and the mix will need to be discarded.

CAUTION: *Dan Shen* **should be avoided in pregnancy, by those taking anticoagulant or antiplatelet drugs, where there is a tendency to bleeding and where the syndrome is not associated with stagnant Blood.**

CHAPTER 8

Growing Sage

Although many of the half-hardy members of the Salvia family from South America and the tropics tend to be grown as annuals in Western Europe, almost all of them are perennials. *Salvia viridis* (painted sage) and *S. plebeia* are the only true annuals listed in chapter 2—all the others are herbaceous perennials or shrubs, and most are fairly tolerant as to soil and growing conditions.

Many members of the family are native to limestone areas and are more than happy on fast-draining, alkaline soil—although, being tolerant creatures, they will grow almost as contentedly in clay.

COMMON SAGE AND OTHER HARDY SHRUBS

Common sage (*S. officinalis*) is a shrubby evergreen. Most sage bushes will grow to around 80cm (32in) in height, with a spread of around 1m (3ft) over three or four years.

If you plan to grow sage for medicinal or culinary use it is best to stay with either common green sage or else the red sage (*S. officinalis* 'Purpurescens Group') traditionally preferred for herbal remedies. The ornamental cultivars listed in chapter 2 retain some of the aroma and therapeutic properties of the original species but tend not to be quite so effective.

Other hardy shrubs that can be grown in the same way include: Greek sage (*S. fruticosa*), Spanish sage (*S. lavandulifolia*), Mexican red bush (*S. microphylla* var. *microphylla*), Jim sage (*S. clevelandii*) and *S. pomifera*.

All these sages originate in warm areas, and although they will survive most northern winters they can be damaged by severe frosts.

Site selection

Choose a sunny, well-drained site, ideally with alkaline to neutral soil. Avoid frost pockets or sites where the plant will catch early morning sun on cold winter dawns. Good drainage is important—sages grown in damp or wet soils are more prone to slug attack, especially Spanish sage which tends to form rosettes of leaves at ground level. Rich soils are likely to encourage foliage rather than flowers, so fresh garden compost should be avoided. Very acid or peat soils should have a lime dressing before planting with sage bushes to help reduce the acidity.

Most sages like bright, sunny places; they will grow in shade if need be, and in hot countries this can actually be preferable, but in Britain and other northern areas as sunny a place as possible is generally best.

Sages are also brittle stemmed and can easily be damaged in high winds. This is especially true of older shrubs which may be completely destroyed in severe weather. Common sage plants tend to become very woody and misshapen after a few years, especially if cropped regularly, so expect to replace the plants every three or four years.

Buying plants

Sage plants are readily available in specialist nurseries, garden centres and even supermarkets. As always when buying nursery-grown plants, look for strong, healthy specimens with plenty of new growth and space in the pot for expansion. Straggly, yellowing herbs will not improve when planted out in the garden, they will simply be a disappointment.

Examine plants for any pests such as red spider mite, aphids and whitefly which can congregate on the undersides of leaves or on new growth and will prove unwelcome additions to a healthy garden.

Most herb nurseries expect a peak in sales in mid- to late spring and gear production to these times. Later in the season plants may have become pot-bound with a mass of tangled roots emerging at the bottom. Good nurseries will regularly pot up their products to larger containers as the season progresses, but then the price of the herbs usually rises accordingly. You can check on roots and potting practices by upturning the pot and tapping gently so that it slides out of the container. Healthy root growth should be evident and the compost should hold its shape. Loose soil suggests that the plant has only recently been potted up and there has been little time to establish the root system.

A convenient and low-cost source of common sage plants can be the supermarket fresh produce display, with clusters of small seedlings sold in pots for kitchen use. These pots are intended simply to sit on the windowsill providing a readily available source of fresh herb over a few weeks, but you can easily pot the baby plants into separate 7.5cm (3in) pots and grow them on in a cool greenhouse or on a windowsill until they are sufficiently estab-lished to be planted out.

The confusion between Greek sage and common sage, men-tioned in earlier chapters, can lead to mislabelling. If in doubt compare the leaf shapes of a red or purple sage plant with one offered as common sage: if the common sage leaves seem narrower or smoother then the odds are that it is really Greek sage. If there are any lobed leaves (see diagram 7) then it most certainly is.

Germination

Like other shrubby herbs common sage can be grown from seed, but germination may be erratic and unless you want dozens of plants in the garden, this is not the most efficient method of culti-

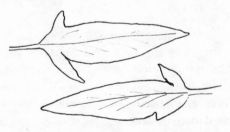

Diagram 7: Trilobed leaves of Greek sage (S. fruticosa)

vation. Sow the seeds in late autumn or spring in a seed tray or 7.5cm (3in) pot containing well watered, good quality compost. Cover the seeds with a fine layer of compost roughly equal in depth to the size of the seed and then cover the tray with glass or place the pot in a plastic bag and store in a warm place (up to about 20°C/68°F).

Germination can occur in two to three weeks but may take longer. As soon as the seedlings are large enough to handle prick them out into a second seed tray, eventually potting on into 7.5cm (3in) pots before hardening off and planting out. With autumn sowings the established sage plants should be ready to plant out in the following spring.

Propagation

Semi-ripe cuttings can be selected from the side shoots in late summer or early autumn, or you can use the new softwood growth in spring and early summer when the root must develop quickly if the cutting is to survive. Cuttings can conveniently be collected when the shrub is pruned after flowering.

Simply break or cut off a suitable shoot, keeping a heel of the main stem attached if possible. Coat the base of the cutting in hormone rooting powder, set half a dozen in good quality compost in a 7.5cm (3in) pot and water well. Leave the pot in a cool greenhouse or cold frame, watering it occasionally, and after a few weeks pot on the rooted cuttings into individual pots, ready for hardening off and planting out in the spring.

Pruning and controlling

Sage is relatively trouble free and regular cutting for culinary or medicinal use will generally keep the plant under control.

Prune after flowering in late summer, cutting back to give 10–15cm (4–6in) new growth. Sage is unlikely to set seed in northern climates, so there is no need to worry about self-seeded plants. Trim back frost-damaged stems in late spring.

HARDY HERBACEOUS PERENNIAL SAGES

In this group come our native sages, *S. pratensis* and wild clary (*S. verbenaca*), as well as North American and Eurasian species like *S. lyrata*, *S. moorcroftiana*, clary sage (*S. sclarea*), *Dan Shen* (*S. miltiorrhiza*) and *S. judaica*. While most of these tend to tolerate cold very well, they don't usually like damp winters so losses are inevitable in our British climate.

Like the shrubby sages these herbaceous perennials are tolerant of a wide range of soils, although as they tend to form basal rosettes of leaves damp areas are best avoided to limit slug damage. Damp soil will also tend to rot the roots—which is the main problem in wet winters. The basal interest of the foliage can make them quite difficult to place in the flower garden: most can be fairly tall when in bloom but for the rest of the season the main interest is at ground level, so they are easily lost among other plants at the back of a bed and can look too large when flowering at the front.

Supports are rarely necessary as the tall flowering stems are usually stiff enough to carry the flowers without bending; like shrubs, wind damage can be a problem in exposed areas. After the first flowers start to wither, cut the stems to ground level to encourage a repeat flowering.

Most of these hardy perennials are grown from seed, sown during spring or early summer in a seed tray containing well watered, good quality compost. Cover the seeds with a fine layer of compost and place on a warm windowsill or in a propagator (at around 20°C/68°F). Germination usually takes 15–20 days.

As soon as the seedlings are large enough to handle, prick them out into 7.5cm (3in) pots before hardening off and planting out in mid- to late summer in a sunny place. The plants will flower the following summer.

Plants like clary sage, wild clary and *S. moorcroftiana* readily self-seed and are often treated as biennials as they die down after flowering and setting seed. Clipping the flowers before the seed sets can preserve the life of the plant. Others, such as *S. lyrata*, can also be propagated by division in the autumn or by cuttings taken in spring.

Seeds and young plants of Chinese red sage or *Dan Shen* are sometimes found in specialist nurseries. The plant prefers moist, sandy soil and will grow to 60cm (2ft) in height. Propagation is by root division in autumn or early spring before the leaves appear. Dig up the root and cut into two or three sections before replanting.

HALF-HARDY HERBACEOUS PERENNIAL SAGES

These plants will generally survive in temperatures down to 0°C (32°F), although some tender varieties will be damaged or destroyed as soon as the temperature drops below 5°C (41°F).

In the half-hardy category are pineapple sage (*S. elegans* 'Scarlet Pineapple'), tangerine sage (*S. elegans*), fruit-scented sage (*S. dorsiana*), and tropical sage (*S. coccinea*). These tend to be treated as container-plants or annuals in Britain and similar northern climates.

Most don't flower until the early autumn, or at best late summer, so they tend to be less commonly grown in British gardens although they are occasionally found in specialist nurseries. Pineapple sage, for example, will happily remain blooming in northern gardens during December and January and its bright scarlet flowers make an attractive feature in winter gardens—until the frosts arrive. In a mild season it will grow to around 2m (6ft), spread to 1m (3ft) and will continue flowering well into early spring.

These tender perennials are best propagated from semi-ripe cuttings in late summer—follow the instructions given on p. 105 for common sage. Over-winter the young cuttings in a cool greenhouse and plant out the following spring when all danger of frosts is over. Because the plant can easily be damaged in a cold winter, always take cuttings in autumn to ensure a supply for the following year. Alternatively, grow on young plants in a container, which can be brought inside when the weather turns cold and are ideal for a conservatory.

ANNUAL SAGES

Painted clary (*S. viridis*) is the only true annual likely to be grown in Britain—the oriental *S. plebeia* is not only tender, but seeds are rarely available. Painted sage is best sown where it is intended to flower on a sunny site, in spring once the last frosts are over and the soil is warm. Germination will take about three weeks and the plant will flower throughout the summer. Ornamental varieties, such as *S. viridis* 'Claryssa', have tiny flowers enclosed in attractive papery bracts in shades of lilac, purple and rose and will flower throughout the summer.

CONTAINER-GROWN SAGE

Young common sage plants are ideal in window boxes and containers for those without a garden. However, most varieties will soon outgrow such sites so will really need replacing every two years. *S. officinalis* 'Tricolor' and 'Icterina' are decorative and will stay small for longer, but they are not fully hardy and lack the strong flavour and therapeutic properties of common or purple sage. Young Greek sage plants will also look good in a container for a couple of years.

Pineapple sage, too, will grow happily in a container, but it is potentially a big bush and soon looks unhappy confined in a pot: transplanting to a very large tub in a conservatory is one solution.

S. viridis 'Claryssa' grows to around 37cm (15in) so can look colourful in a large container for patio or terrace. Others suitable for container growing include: *S. coccinea* and *S. microphylla*.

As always for container-plants, regular feeding is important, preferably with a liquid feed or with fertiliser sticks inserted in the compost. Pinching out the growing tops will also help to keep the plants compact and bushy.

CHAPTER 9

Cooking with Sage

Like many traditional culinary herbs sage is excellent for the digestion, so using it in cooking not only adds a delicious flavour, but also helps digestive function. It is a carminative, so helps to reduce stomach gases, leading to flatulence, and as a bitter remedy also stimulates the digestive processes.

In traditional Galenic medicine its dry, warming nature (hot in the third degree according to some early writers) would also have made it an ideal counterbalance to cold and damp foods. It would have been seen as an ideal flavouring for 'windy' vegetables like beans or to combat the chills that may accompany too much fish.

Today, we mainly use sage in cooking to improve the digestion of fatty foods or those that are difficult to digest. In many parts of Southern Europe it is still customary to cover joints of pork and veal with sage leaves when roasting them: both are difficult meats to digest, so the addition of sage is a practical way of flavouring the dish and supporting digestive function. In Britain it was traditionally used with fatty meats like duck and goose—no doubt the origin of our traditional habit of eating sage and onion stuffing with the Christmas poultry. In Germany and Belgium sage is a traditional accompaniment to eels which are equally difficult to digest.

However, it is worth remembering the advise of one French chef (Palaiseul, 1973) and not 'over-egg' the dish with other herbs—'In the grand opera of cooking, sage represents an easily-offended prima donna. It likes to have the stage almost to itself . . .' Sage really is best used by itself and not included in a bouquet garni with thyme or marjoram or even helped with a little parsley or chervil like many other herbs. Its strong flavour is, however, very useful for transforming mundane dishes into something special—meatballs or burgers made from minced meat and onions always taste significantly better for a little sage. Chopped sage is good added to pastry for both savoury and sweet tarts and pies—it goes especially well with apple tarts—and sage also transforms cheese sandwiches. You can use it instead of basil in pesto or add a couple of small leaves to cabbage or broad bean dishes. Sage was also traditionally used to flavour cheeses and is still found in Sage Derby, for example. Walsh's *Manual of Domestic Economy* from 1857 gives suitable instructions for enthusiastic cheese-makers (quoted by Mrs Grieve, 1931):

> Bruise the tops of young red Sage on a mortar with some leaves of spinach and squeeze the juice; mix it with the rennet in the milk, more or less, according to the preferred colour and taste. When the curd is come, break it gently and put it in with the skimmer till it is pressed two inches above the vat. Press it 8 or 10 hours. Salt it and turn every day.

Sage mustard is also very useful to keep in the kitchen: process a handful of sage leaves in a small food blender, then add 1–2 tablespoons of Dijon mustard and blend well. Store the mustard in a small jar in the refrigerator. It is good added to stir-fried chicken with *crème fraîche* or used as a garnish for home-cooked ham or grilled pork chops.

Sage has been used for centuries with onions in sauces and stuffings. A recipe given by Mrs Grieve (1931), taken from *The Cook's Oracle* of 1821, is for a sauce:

> Chop very fine an ounce of onion and ½oz of green Sage leaves, put them in a stamper with 4 spoonsful of water, simmer gently for 10 minutes, then put in a teaspoonful of pepper and salt and 1oz of fine breadcrumbs. Mix well together, then pour to it ¼pt of Broth, Gravy or Melted Butter, stir well together and simmer a few minutes longer. This is a relishing sauce for Roast Pork, Goose or Duck, or with Green Peas on Meagre Days.

Sage also makes a good substitute for cinnamon when making mulled wine. You can make sage wine by steeping a large mugful of leaves in 75cl (26½fl oz) of dry white wine for ten days. Pour off the wine, sweeten with a little honey and use as an apéritif before lunch or dinner. The unsweetened wine can also be used in cooking.

Sue Lawrence, in *Feasting on Herbs* (1995), gives a good recipe for sage jelly which enthusiastic jam-makers might like to try. It is made by cooking 1.25kg (3lb) of cooking apples with 900ml (1½pts) of water and 25g (1oz) of sage leaves. After about 40 minutes, when the apples are soft and pulpy, add 600ml (1pt) of distilled clear vinegar and then drip the pulp through a jelly bag (suspended from an upturned stool and scalded with boiling water) and leave it for up to 24 hours. The clear jelly is then reheated gently with sugar (500g/1lb to every 600ml/1pt of liquid) until the sugar has dissolved before being boiled rapidly until the setting point is reached. Remove from the heat and stir in 25g (1oz) of finely chopped sage leaves before potting in warmed jars.

The flavours of the different species can also be very variable. Many find common sage rather predominant, but Greek or Spanish sage can be rather more subtle—as can the various variegated *S. officinalis* cultivars (see p. 26) which also look very decorative on a dish.

Saltimbocca

This traditional Italian dish is usually made by rolling a flattened veal escalope and a slice of Parma ham tightly together around one or two sage leaves. This sometimes seems to make the sage—especially fresh sage leaves in summer—rather too dominant, so try this version instead:

Use one flattened veal escalope, one sage leaf and one slice of Parma ham per person. Fold both escalope and ham in half and then interleave them with the sage leaf in the middle to form a flat, loosely folded, square parcel of four alternating layers of meat. There is no need to tie the parcels with string or fix with a cocktail stick. Dust with seasoned flour and set aside.

Sauté a finely chopped onion in 1–2 tablespoons of olive oil. Then sauté your meat parcels for 2–3 minutes each side until the meat is tender and cooked through. Place in a warm serving dish and keep hot.

Add 1 dessertspoon of flour to the onions remaining in the pan and stir thoroughly while continuing to heat for 2-3 minutes. Then add 2 tablespoons of marsala, stir well, and add 150ml (¼pt) of chicken stock. Continue heating and stirring until the sauce thickens; season with freshly ground sea salt and black pepper as required, then pour over the escalopes and serve immediately.

It goes well with rice and green salad or new boiled potatoes and French beans. Flattened pork escalopes can be used instead of veal if preferred.

Saltimbocca of red mullet

A delicious alternative, suggested by the chef Alistair Little (Little and Whittington, 1993), is to use red mullet fillets instead of veal. He inevitably uses fresh red mullet which needs to be pin-boned with tweezers. My cheat is to use frozen red mullet fillets.

Allow two frozen fillets and two small slices of Parma ham per person. When the fillets have thawed place a very thin sliver of butter on the flesh side and wrap butter and fish with a Parma ham slice. Place a sage leaf on the outer skin side of each fish parcel and set aside in the refrigerator for 30–60 minutes.

When ready to cook, dust the parcels in seasoned flour on both sides. Melt 25g (1oz) of butter in a frying-pan and sauté the red mullet parcels for 2–3 minutes each side, starting with the flesh side. Place on a warm serving dish and discard any cooking juices from the pan but do not wipe it. Return the pan to the heat and cook 25g (1oz) of butter until it just starts to brown and foam. Then add the juice of 1 lemon, stir well and pour the foaming mixture over the fish. This is one dish that really must be served immediately—the sauce goes unpleasantly greasy if it is kept hot for any time.

The mullet saltimbocca goes well in summer with boiled mixed young seasonal vegetables—baby potatoes, carrots, broad beans, mangetout and thin asparagus tips—and is equally good with just green salad and boiled pink fir potatoes.

Calves' liver with sage

Another traditional Italian dish is to serve calves' liver with sage and onions. Again recipes vary enormously but a simple one is as follows:

Thinly slice a large onion or two medium-sized ones (for four people). Melt 50g (2oz) of butter (or 25g/1oz of butter and 1 tablespoon of olive oil if you prefer) in a large frying-pan and cook the onions very slowly over a low heat—it will take about 30 minutes and the onions should be soft and golden. Add one sage leaf per person to the onions after about 20 minutes of cooking.

Use one thin slice of calves' liver per person. Place the liver on top of the onions, raise the heat and cook for 2–3 minutes each side. The liver should be soft and slightly pink; if you prefer it well done then cook for longer. Put the liver and most of the onions into a warm serving plate and keep warm. Add 1 dessertspoon of balsam vinegar and a small glass of red wine to the saucepan and boil vigorously so that the wine thickens. Season with salt and freshly ground black pepper and pour over the liver. Serve immediately.

This dish goes well with boiled new potatoes, mangetout and peas.

Stuffed mushrooms with sage

These make a pleasant starter or lunch dish. Use one or two large flat cap or Portabellini mushrooms per person—wipe, trim and set aside in a shallow baking dish.

To stuff six mushrooms you will need one finely chopped, medium-sized onion, a crushed clove of garlic, 2 heaped tablespoons of wholemeal breadcrumbs, 1 heaped tablespoon of grated cheddar, two more of the mushrooms, finely chopped, and three large finely chopped sage leaves.

Sauté the onion and garlic in 1 tablespoon of olive oil, then add the mushrooms and continue cooking until they soften. Add the breadcrumbs, sage and cheese and mix well.

Put a spoonful of the stuffing mixture onto each flat mushroom in the dish and then bake for 10–15 minutes (200°C/400°F/Gas mark 6). Serve on a bed of green salad with a French dressing.

Pasta with sage and courgettes

Ideally you need a tiny boat-shaped pasta for this dish but small shells work just as well.

One medium-sized courgette, a cup of pasta and three finely chopped sage leaves are enough for two people for lunch. Cut the courgettes into matchstick-size pieces and sauté in a tablespoon of olive oil for 3–4 minutes or until they just start to soften. Add the chopped sage and a crushed clove of garlic. Cook for 2–3 minutes more and remove from the heat.

Meanwhile, cook the pasta (fresh or dried) in salted boiling water as directed on the packet. When it is ready, strain the pasta and add the courgette mixture, plus 2 teaspoons of freshly grated Parmesan cheese and freshly ground black pepper. Toss well and drizzle over a little olive oil. Serve with a green salad for lunch or by itself as a starter.

Cooking with clary sage

As well as using clary sage (*S. sclarea*) to flavour and enhance wines and ales (see p. 28), the leaves were traditionally made into fritters or added to pancakes.

Make a fairly thick batter from flour, eggs and milk in the usual way (the sort of consistency used for Yorkshire pudding is ideal). Choose good-sized clary leaves and wash them carefully, patting dry on kitchen paper. Dip the leaves into the batter mix and fry in butter until they are crisp, then serve at once with fresh lemon juice or maple syrup if preferred.

Cooking with pineapple sage

Pineapple sage (*S. elegans* 'Scarlet Pineapple') is also well worth using in the kitchen. Add a sprig of the plant to a bottle of sparkling water, close the bottle lid tightly and leave for 3–5 days to give a hint of pineapple to the drink. A sprig added to apple or elderflower cordials before serving also gives an interesting flavour.

The chopped leaves are good added to sweet pastry for a pineapple flan: add 1 tablespoon of finely chopped leaves per 100g (4oz) of flour, using your favourite pastry recipe, and bake the flan blind. Then fill the flan case with layers of chopped fresh pineapple and whipped cream or *crème fraîche*. Decorate with small whole leaves.

A few whole leaves placed in the bottom of a sponge cake tin before adding the sponge mixture also give a good flavour to the sponge. They work well with fruit salads, too—either added on their own or with chopped pineapple or ginger mint.

For savoury dishes, make pineapple sage mustard (as for sage, p. 110) or add to caramelised onions as a garnish.

Slowly sauté 2–3 thinly sliced red onions in 2 tablespoons of olive oil for about 30 minutes until they are soft and golden. Add a tablespoon of balsamic vinegar and a heaped tablespoon of finely chopped pineapple sage leaves and a pinch of sugar. Stir well and cook for a further 5 minutes until the mixture is well blended. Serve hot with grilled pork chops or gammon, or cold with ham and salads.

Glossary

Adrenal cortex—part of the adrenal gland located above the kidneys, which produces several steroidal hormones.

Alkaloid—active plant constituent containing nitrogen and which usually has a significant effect on bodily function.

Anthelmintic—destroys parasitic worms.

Antihidrotic—reduces body secretions, including sweat and saliva.

Antioxidant—a substance which delays the degradation of chemical oxidation.

Antispasmodic—reduces muscle spasm and tension.

Astringent—used to describe a herb which will precipitate proteins from the surface of cells or membranes, causing tissues to contract and tighten; forms a protective coating and stops bleeding and discharges.

Bract—a floral leaf.

Calyx—the outer whorl of floral leaves.

Carminative—expels gas from the stomach and intestines to relieve flatulence, digestive colic and gastric discomfort.

Demulcent—softens and soothes damaged or inflamed surfaces, such as the gastric mucous membranes.

Depurative—blood purifier.

Diaphoretic—increases sweating.

Diuretic—encourages urine flow.

Emmenagogue—stimulates menstrual flow.

Expectorant—enhances the secretion of sputum from the respiratory tract so that it is easier to cough up.

Flavonoids—active plant constituents which improve the circulation and may also have diuretic, anti-inflammatory and antispasmodic effects.

Free radical—group of atoms capable of free existence under special conditions for short periods; they contain unpaired electrons and are highly reactive.

Hyperglycaemic—increases blood sugar levels.

Hypertensive—raises blood pressure.

Hypoglycaemic—reduces blood sugar levels.

Hypotensive—lowers blood pressure.

Inflorescence—method in which flowers are arranged on an axis.

Lanceolate—slightly broad or tapering to a point; lance-shaped.

Lyrate—lyre-shaped.

Menorrhagia—abnormally heavy menstrual bleeding.

Mucilage/mucilaginous—a plant containing complex sugar molecules that are soft and slippery and provide protection for the mucous membranes and inflamed surfaces.

Nervine—herb that affects the nervous system and which may be stimulating or sedating.

Ovate—egg-shaped leaves attached at the broader end.

Peripheral vasodilator—relaxes peripheral blood vessels supplying to the limbs, skin and muscles (including heart muscles).

Parasympathetic nervous system—a subdivision of the autonomic nervous system, also known as the craniosacral system. The action of these nerves is to slow down activity in the glands and smooth muscles which they supply.

Raceme—inflorescence having a common axis with stalked flowers developing successively along it so that the youngest are at the apex.

Qi (ch'i)—the body's vital energy as defined in Chinese medicine.

Styptic—stops external bleeding.

Tannin—active plant constituents which are astringent and combine with proteins. The term is derived from plants used in tanning leather.

Thujones—toxic terpenoid ketones found in some varieties of sage.

Vermifuge—destroys parasitic worms.

Vulnerary—wound herb.

Xue—Blood, one of the fundamental substances in Chinese medicine.

Useful Addresses

The United Kingdom
Professional herbal organisations
The General Council and Register of Consultant Herbalists, Marlborough House, Swanpool, Falmouth, Cornwall TR11 4HW.
National Institute of Medical Herbalists, 56 Longbrook Street, Exeter, Devon EX4 6AH.
The Register of Chinese Herbal Medicine, 19 Trinity Road, London N2 8JJ.

Mail order herb suppliers
G. Baldwin & Co, 171–174 Walworth Road, London SE17 1RW.
East West Herbs Ltd., Langston Priory Mews, Kingham, Oxon OX7 6UW.
Hambledon Herbs, Court Farm, Milverton, Somerset TA4 1NF.
Neal's Yard Remedies, 26–34 Ingate Place, London SW8 3NS.

Nurseries and specialist plant suppliers
Cheshire Herbs, Fourfields, Forest Road, Little Budworth, Tarporeley, Cheshire CW6 9ES.
Chiltern Seeds, Bortree Stile, Ulverston, Cumbria LA12 7PB.
Iden Croft Herbs, Frittenden Road, Staplehurst, Kent TN12 0DN.
Poyntzfield Herb Nursery, Black Isle, By Dingwall. Ross and Cromarty IV7 8LX.

The USA
Associations
American Botanical Council, PO Box 210660, Austin, TX 78720. Tel: (512) 331-8868.
American Herbal Products Association, PO Box 2410, PO Box 210660, Austin, TX 78720. Tel: (512) 331-8555.

USEFUL ADDRESSES

The American Herbalists' Guild, PO Box 1683, Soquel, CA 95073.
Tel: (408) 464-2441.
Northeast Herb Association, PO Box 266, Milton, NY 12547.
The Herb Research Federation, 1007 Pearl Street, Suite 500, Boulder, CO 808302.

Suppliers
Bay Laurel Farm, West Garzas Road, Camel Valley, CA 93924.
Tel: (408) 659-2913.
Frontier, Box 299, Norway, Iowa 52318. Tel: (800) 669-3275.
May Way Trading Chinese Herb Company, 1338 Cypress Street, Oakland, CA 94607. Tel: (510) 208-3113.
Herbs Products Co, 11012 Magnolia Blvd., North Hollywood, CA 91601. Tel: (818) 984-3141.
Kiehls Pharmacy, 109 Third Avenue, New York, NY10009.
Sage Mountain Herbs, PO Box 420, East Barre, VT 05649. Tel: (802) 479-9825.

References and Further Reading

Ambastha, S. P. (ed.) (1986). *The Useful Plants of India*, CSIR, New Delhi.

Alzheimer's Disease Society News (1997). Research report, May 1997.

Arano, L. C. (1976). *Tacuinum Sanitatis*, Electa Editrice, Milan; trs. O. Ratti and A. Westbrook as *The Mediaeval Health Handbook*, George Braziller, New York.

Beckham, N. (1995). *Menopause: A positive approach using natural therapies*, Viking, Victoria.

Bensky, S., and Gamble, A. (1986). *Chinese Herbal Medicine*, Eastland Press, Seattle.

Bone, K. (1996). *Clinical Applications of Chinese and Ayurvedic Herbs*, Phytotherapy Press, Queensland.

Brieskorn, C. (1991). *Z. Phytotherapie*, **12**, 61–9.

Brieskorn, C., and Biechele, W. (1971). *Arch. Pharm.*, **304**, 557–61.

Brieskorn, C., and Dalferth, S. (1864). *Deutsch. Apoth. Ztg.*, **106**, 1388–92.

Brieskorn, C., and Dömling, H. J. (1969). *Arch. Pharm.*, **302**, 641–5.

Brieskorn, C., and Kapadia, Z. (1979). *Planta Medica*, **35**, 376–8.

Brieskorn, C., and Kapadia, Z. (1980). *Planta Medica*, **38**, 86–90.

Brook, R. (*c.* 1830). *A New Family Herbal*, pub. R. Brook, Huddersfield.

Cabo, J., *et al.* (1985). *Ars Pharmaceutica*, **26**, 239–49.

Chang, H., and But, P. (1986). *Pharmacology and Applications of Chinese Materia Medica*, vol. 1, World Scientific, Singapore.

Chevallier, A. (1996). *The Encyclopedia of Medicinal Plants*, Dorling Kindersley, London.

Chiba, K., Takakuwa, T., Tada, M., and Yoshii, T. (1992). *Biosci. Biotech. Biochem.*, **56**, 1769–72.

Croteau, R., El-Bialy, H., and El-Hindawi, S. (1984). *Arch. Biochem. Biophys.*, **228**, 667–80.

Culpeper, N. (1653). *Complete Herbal and English Physician*, London; 1826 edition published by J. Gleave, Manchester.

Davis, P. (1988). *Aromatherapy: An A–Z*, C. W. Daniel, Saffron Walden.

van der Dries, J. A. A., and Baerheim Svendsen, A. A. (1989). *Flavour Fragrance Journal*, **4**, 59–61.

Duke. J. A. (1983). *Medicinal Plants of the Bible*, Trado-Medic Books, Owerri, NY.

Duke, J. A. (1997). *Herbs for Health*, November/December 1997; summarised in *Greenfiles*, Spring 1998, 17.

van Dyke, T. E., Braswell, L., and Offenbacher, S. (1986). *Agents and Actions*, **19**, 376–7.

European Scientific Cooperative on Phytotherapy (1996). Monograph on Salviae Folium, in *ESCOP Fascicule 2*, March 1996.

Foster, S., and Chongxi, Y. (1992). *Herbal Emissaries*, Healing Arts Press, Rochester, Vermont.

Fox, L. (1999). Herbal Remedies of Myddfai: Remnants of Druid lore?, *Herbs*, **24** (3), 19–21.

Franchomme, P. (1985). *Advanced therapy for infectious diseases*, International Phytomedical Foundation, France; Seminar on Germicidal Oils, November 24–25, 1985, London.

Fratkin, K. (1986). *Chinese Herbal Patent Formulas*, Shya Publications, Boulder, Colorado.

Frawley, D., and Lad, V. (1988). *The Yoga of Herbs*, Lotus Press, Santa Fe.

Gattefossé, R.-M. (1937). *Aromatherapie*; trs. R. Tisserand as *Gattefossé's Aromatherapy* (1993), C. W. Daniel, Saffron Walden.

Gerard, J. (1597). *The Herball or General Historie of Plants*, John Norton, London.

Goodyer, J. (1655). *Dioscorides' Materia Medica*, ed. R. T. Gunther (1933), Oxford University Press, Oxford.

Gracza, L., and Ruff, P. (1984). *Arch. Pharm.*, **317**, 339–45.

Grieve, M. (1931). *A Modern Herbal*, Jonathan Cape, London.

Guo, S. K. *et al.*, (1983). *Planta Medica*, **48**, 63.

Halliwell, B. *et al.* (1995). *Food Chemical Toxicology*, **33** (7), 601–17.

Herbs for Health (1988). Sage, rosemary, balm and more—the latest research on Alzheimer's, *Herbs for Health*, Jan/Feb 1998, 48–51.

Hilan, C., Khazzakha, K., and Sfeir, R. (1997). *The British Journal of Phytotherapy*, **4**, 155–62.

Holmes, P. (1989). *The Energetics of Western Herbs*, Artemis Press, Boulder, Colorado.

Hort, A. (trs.) (1916). *Theophrastus's Enquiry into Plants*, Loeb's Classical Library, William Heinemann, London.

Itzhaki, J. (1995). When sage may be the wisest remedy, *New Scientist*, 14 October 1996, 10.

Jalsenjak, V., Peljnjak, S., and Kustrak, D. (1987). *Pharmazie*, **42**, 419–20.

Janssen, A. M. (1989). *Antimicrobial activities of essential oils—a pharmacognistical study* (Dissertation), Rijkuniversiteit te Leiden, 91–108.

Jones, W. H. S. (trs.) (1951). *Pliny's Natural History*, vols. 6 and 7, Loeb's Classical Library, William Heinemann, London.

Keji, C. (1981). *Am. J. Chinese Med.*, **9**, 193.

Lawrence, S. (1995). *Feasting on Herbs*, Kyle Cathie, London.

Li, D. *et al.* (1987). *Henan J. of TCM*, **1**, 29; English abstract *Traditional Chinese Medicine Digest*, **2**, (3–4), 41 (1987).

Li, N.-H. (ed.), (1985). *Chinese Medicinal Herbs of Hong Kong*, vol. 4, Chinese Medical Research Institute, Hong Kong.

Liao *et al.* (1987). *Sichuanxhongui*, **5**, 18; English abstract *Abstracts on Chinese Medicine*, **2**, 336 (1988).

Lin, Z. (1983). *Hubei J. of TCM*, **3**, 9; English abstract *Traditional Chinese Medicine Digest*, **1** (2), 37 (1987).

Little, A., and Whittington, R. (1993). *Alistair Little: Keep it Simple*, Conran Octopus, London.

Lo, A. C. *et al.* (1992). *Eur. J. Drug. Metab. Pharmacokin.*, **17**, 257.

Mabberley, D. J. (1987). *The Plant Book*, Cambridge University Press, Cambridge.

Mabey, R. (1996). *Flora Britannica*, Sinclair-Stevenson, London.

Maciocia, G. (1995). *The Three Treasures*, Paeony Press, London.

Mailhebiau, P. (1995). *Portraits in Oils*, C. W. Daniel, Saffron Walden.

Müller, J., Köll-Weber, M., and Kraus, W. (1992). *Planta Medica*, **58** (Suppl. I), A678.

Murko, D. *et al.* (1974). *Planta Medica*, **25**, 295.

Nakatani, N. (1994). Antioxidative and antimicrobial constituents of herbs and spices, *Spices, Herbs and Edible Fungi*, Elsevier Science, Amsterdam, 251-71.

Newall, C., Anderson, L. A., and Phillipson, J. D. (1996). *Herbal Medicines*, Pharmaceutical Press, London.

Palaiseul, J. (1973). *Grandmother's Secrets*, Barrie & Jenkins, London.

Petri, G. *et al.* (1988). *Planta Medica*, **54**, 575.

Pughe, J. (1861). *The Herbal Remedies of the Physicians of Myddfai*, reprinted Llanerch Enterprises, Lampeter, 1987.

Quincy, J. (1724). *Pharmacopoeia Officinalis & Extemporanea or The Complete English Dispensatory*, E. Bell, London.

Rösing, R. J. (1989). *Sweatosan-Studie*, unpublished: quoted in *ESCOP* (1996).

Rovesti, P., and Gattefossé, H. M. (1973). *Labo-Pharma. Probl. Techn.*, **223**, 32–8.

Rutherford, D. M. *et al.* (1992). *Neuroscience Letters*, **135**, 224–6.

Schauenberg, P., and Paris, F. (1974). *Guide to Medicinal Plants*, Delachaux & Niestle, Neuchatel; English edition 1977, Lutterworth Press, London.

Sharman, P., and Billing, J. (1998). *Quarterly Review of Biology*, March 1998.

Sinclair Rohde, E. (1922). *The Old English Herbals*, Longman Green, London.

Singh, U., Wadhani, A. M., and Johri, B. M. (1983). *Dictionary of Economic Plants of India*, Indian Council of Agricultural Research, New Delhi.

Steinegger, E., and Hänsel, R. (1992). *Pharmakognosie*, Springer, Berlin.

Sutton, J. (1999). *The Gardener's Guide to Growing Salvias*, David & Charles, Newton Abbot.

Svoboda, K. P., and Deans, S. G. (1990). *Variability of rosemary and sage volatile oils obtained from plants of various geographical sources and antioxidative properties of solvent extracts*, 21st International Symposium on Essential Oils, Lahti, Finland.

Taddei, I. *et al.* (1988). *Fitoterapia*, **59**, 463–8.

Takácsova, M., Pribela, A., and Faktorová, M. (1995). *Nahrung*, **39**(3), 241–3.

Tisserand, R. (1977). *The Art of Aromatherapy*, C. W. Daniel, Saffron Walden.

Turner, W. (1562). *A New Herball*, part 2; facsimile edition of parts 2 and 3 (1568), ed. G. T. L. Chapman, F. McCombie and A. Wesencraft, Cambridge University Press, 1995.

Valnet, J. (1964). *Aromathérapie*, Maloine, Paris.

Vogel, V. J. (1970). *American Indian Medicine*, University of Oklahoma Press, Norman.

Wagner, H. *et al.* (1984). *Plant Drug Analysis*, Springer, Heidelberg.

Wang, F. (1987). *Liaoning J. of TCM*, **3**, 17; English abstract in *Traditional Chinese Medicine Digest*, **2** (1-2), 43 (1987).

Wang, N. *et al.* (1989). *Planta Medica*, **55**, 390.

Weiss, R. J. (1991). *Lehrbuch der Phytotherapie*, 7th ed., Hippokrates Verlag, Stuttgart; the 6th ed. is available in English as *Herbal Medicine*, Beaconsfield Publishers, Beaconsfield.

Wichtl, M. (1989). Salbeiblätter, *Teedrogen* (ed. M. Wichtl), Wiss Verlagsgesellschaft, Stuttgart

Yanchi. L. (1988). *The Essential Book of Traditional Chinese Medicine*, vol. 1: Theory, Columbia University Press, New York.

Yang, S.-Z. (trs.) (1998). *The Divine Farmer's Materia Medica: a translation of the Shen Nong Ben Cao Jing*, Blue Poppy Press, Boulder, Colarado.

Yehia, A., and Marth, E. H. (1993). *Journal of Food Protection*, **56**, 876–8.

REFERENCES AND FURTHER READING

Yen, K.-Y. (1992). *The Illustrated Chinese Materia Medica*, SMC Publishing, Taipei.

Yeung, H.-C. (1985). *Handbook of Chinese Herbs and Formulae*, vol. 1, Institute of Chinese Medicine, Los Angeles.

Zhang, X. *et al.* (1982). *J. of New TCM*, **3**, 27; English abstract in *Traditional Chinese Medicine Digest*, **1** (1), 31.

Zhu, B. *et al.* (1987). *Chinese Journal Integrated. Traditional and Western Medicine*, **7**, 591.